STRESSORS AND COPING
STRATEGIES FOR DAILY LIVING

Books published by
Bright Destiny Osaiyuwu

A Perilous Escape from Africa
Trudeau and The Hunter's Rabbit
Animals in The Volga Forest

STRESSORS AND COPING
STRATEGIES FOR DAILY LIVING

Advice for a Healthier Life

Bright Destiny Osaiyuwu

To my beloved mother, Mrs. Vero Omoregie Osaiyuwu.

CONTENTS

Introduction

THIS BOOK IS about the things that cause stress, the different coping strategies people use in coping with stress, and recommended, good coping strategies for these stressors.

Stress is generally defined as what we experience physically, mentally, emotionally, and psychologically. In today's world, stress can be experienced from the environment in which we live, and in our body and thoughts. Stress is inevitable and not something we can always avoid because it is part of life; it is like a killer disease that has ravaged many lives around the globe.

Much of what is happening in the world today has destabilized many people in different ways, causing them stress. There are several negative things stress can do to our wellbeing. Stress can ruin our day and bring out the worst in us; it can destroy what we have built; it can negatively impact everyone around us.

Stress can make people do what they would not normally do. Coping with stress can be challenging, but finding the right coping strategies can help us properly deal with it. When you look around sometimes, you will notice that many people use different coping strategies that they believe will help them cope with their stress. Some smoke cigarettes, some drink alcohol, some use dangerous drugs, and some have other deadly habits.

Before indulging in such negative coping strategies, we should always ask ourselves these questions:

- Are these coping strategies really helping our situation?
- Are these habits helping us contribute positively to our community?
- Are we influencing our children in a positive way?
- What message are we sending those who look up to us?

There are numerous things that can easily stress us out on a daily basis, but before we elaborate on those things, let's look at the causes of stress as well as good, effective coping strategies we can use to manage them.

Chapter One
DEATH OF A LOVED ONE

ONE OF THE causes of intense stress is losing a loved one. When people lose their loved ones, they tend to feel the worst pain of their lives. If they are not careful, that singular occurrence could change their lives forever. So, it is always imperative for us to apply wisdom at this point in time and totally surrender our situation to God in prayers.

Losing a loved one is one of the worst situations anyone could ever experience. That is why when there is a death in the family, other family members, our friends, our colleagues and other well-wishers and sympathizers gather at our homes to give their condolences and support. Expressing their condolences and support is a way to ease the pains of the bereaved.

People's support at that time will give the bereaved

family hope to be able to bear the pains and agonies. After the bereaved bury their loved ones, that is when they will began to stress even more. You may ask why they will be stressed *after* the burial. Well, there are many things that will trigger their moods and thereby make them stress. Their moods will also be affected by the memories of the good deeds of their deceased family member.

What they feel at that time is like post-traumatic stress disorder (PTSD); although it might not be the same, but the emotional states have some similarities. During a time of intense grieving, people who cannot deal with stress may resign themselves to one or more of the bad coping strategies mentioned earlier—for example, smoking or excessive drinking of alcohol as well as other deadly habits. The time of loss and after the funeral process is often the testing period when people can easily fall into wrong coping strategies.

Bear in mind that after this testing period, when people are more in control of their impulses, they are less likely to exhibit such bad coping strategies. Coping with stress after losing people close to our hearts is the most difficult thing to do. That is why we all must play our roles in the best way we can, to support those who have lost the people they love and cherish including putting them in prayers.

Good coping strategies

There are several ways of coping when we lose someone close to our hearts. This is not to say that coping with such a tragic loss is easy; of course, there are some negative effects that naturally come to us when such things happen to us. We feel sad, we cry, and even become aggressive sometimes.

The most effective coping strategies to use after losing a loved one is to pray to God for strength and fortitude to bear the loss as well as to reflect on their positive impact on us and everyone around them while they were alive. Then, we must acknowledge and accept that they are gone; there is no point to been in denial over their death. Stop flogging yourself, trying to hide under the belief that they are still alive or will wake up soon. When we do not accept the fact that they are dead, we are likely daydream and deny their passing, which could increase our stress level. Even after accepting that they are gone, try using their positive deeds to still feel their presence in your life. Knowing how good they were to you can give you the assurance that they are now in a better place, far from this sinful world.

We cry when we miss their presence. When we cry, we tend to feel better afterwards. When we repress crying and grieving—natural responses to the shock of hearing of the death of a loved one—the psychological effects can be detrimental to our health. It is okay to cry after hearing of the death of a loved one because it releases the burden of stress within us and makes us feel better.

Whenever you see anyone crying after losing their loved one, allow them to cry because that is one of the best ways they can mentally and psychologically handle the stress that comes with it. With this in mind, we must also acknowledge that there are people who do not feel like crying after such an incident. It is not that they don't feel the shock or miss the departed soul—they just handle loss in a different way.

Oftentimes, such people cry and bleed in their hearts over the loss. Sometimes they feel the pain more than other family members. However, crying without any physical signs of tears can be more detrimental to their mental health. It feels better to let those tears out rather than keeping and suppressing them inside. Overall, crying is one of the best ways to cope with the stress of losing a loved one.

Another way of coping with the stress of losing a loved one is by hugging family members, friends, or anyone sympathetic to our situation. Many people think that hugging someone is only for fun, but when people hug us, they also show us how much affection they have for us during our difficult time. Knowing that we are not alone in our predicament and that people are there to show their support and love can dramatically reduce our stress level, which will enable us to cope properly.

Losing a loved one can cause a lifetime of pain, sorrow, and agony for many families. There are many who weep on daily basis because of the death of their loved ones. Crying and weeping for the departed souls every day can affect our wellbeing and mental health. It is okay to weep and cry occasionally, but doing it on daily basis is not good for our health.

There are some things people do subconsciously that trigger their moods every day and make them cry over their loved ones daily. Things like leaving pictures of their departed loved ones on their social media platforms, keeping their picture in an open place where they can easily stumble on them, or drawing tattoos of them on their skin.

Let us elaborate more on social media a bit. When pictures of your departed loved ones are left on social media, people are going to comment on the photos. And when they do, it will trigger your mood and possibly spoil your day because you will not be happy seeing those comments; it is like reopening and bruising your old wounds.

When you do these things, you create an avenue of sadness in your life. This is not to say that you shouldn't keep things that will make you remember your loved ones, but there are other ways you can keep their pictures or belongings in such a way that you don't stumble on them on a daily basis. For example, you can print their pictures and keep them in a safe place where you do not have to see them every day.

Put those pictures where they are not too exposed to you. Any time you choose to go to where they are kept to see them, is okay to cry in that moment. Keeping these things hidden doesn't stop people from remembering their loved ones daily; they are still in their subconscious minds anyways. However, putting the photos away will definitely limit the number of times they cry and weep over their departed loved ones. So, it is very important to use these strategies for coping with stress after losing a loved one.

You can talk to people around you who are sympathetic to your situation, people you believe can revive you emotionally. Do not keep everything to yourself; let your thoughts out so that they can contribute positively to your healing process. It is when people suppress these feelings that many of them end up using bad coping strategies or going into depression.

Attune yourself to reality of life and accept the fact that everybody will one day leave this earth. Accept that dying is part of life. Always have the positive belief that your departed loved one is in a better place. Never wish to trade anything in exchange for their life—acknowledge that death is inevitable. By the time you sink these positive thoughts into your head, your stress level will drastically reduce.

Sometimes, reading a book alone about how you can cope with the stress of losing a loved one may not completely get you out of your grieving moments. It is not always guaranteed that the above coping strategies will work for everyone because people react to things differently. If at any time you feel that these coping strategies mentioned above are aggravating your stress level in one way or the other, or not working for you, you can always seek one-on-one professional help from a counsellor or psychologist who can help you get through this difficult time.

Above all, take your situation to God in prayer. Always remember that prayer changes things and that God is the only one who can give you healing and inner peace to recover from your tragic loss.

Chapter Two
ABUSE

LET US LOOK into the stressor of abuse. This kind of stressor has affected so many families around the world. The effects of abuse can be life-changing and can have huge negative impact on the people going through it. Abuse can be experienced in different forms; it could be physical or emotional or both. However, the most difficult to detect is emotional abuse because it is something we experience internally. Abuse does not only happen to women; it equally happens to men too. Reactions to abuse varies, depending on the individual.

Some people react to abuse less, while others react to it in more intense ways. Note that abuse always have negative effects on people; there is nothing positive about it. When someone is going through abuse, there are lots of negativity that goes with it. For example, they will begin to show fear, low self-esteem, anger, aggression, feelings of self-hate, and will start to isolate or withdraw themselves from others. Some will even categorize a particular gender or race as bad just because they had that awful experience with a particular person who fits into those categories.

If a young child has parents who are going through abuse, their grades will begin to drop drastically and other activities in their school will be affected as well. Even if they are not directly abused, it will still affect them in one negative way or the other, especially their performance in school and friendships with their peers. So, abuse has all kinds of negativity attached to it either directly or indirectly.

Let us look at another example: When a woman or man is going through abuse, their child or children are right there witnessing the scenario. Some people may think that young children don't know anything yet. But regardless of their age, as long as they can see, hear, feel, and talk, they will be negatively impacted. Abuse is like a virus that spreads to the things around it. Thinking that young children know nothing about abuse is not a good move because whatever they see, they do.

Abuse can cause traumatic stress during and after it occurs. The abused person may start to experience reflections from it, recalling things like yelling, threats to their life, pushing and pulling, sounds of slammed doors, and other things that may have occurred between the abuser and the abused. These negative reactions can have a huge impact on their lives and can be detrimental to their health and how they function in their day-to-day life. Some people might easily overcome an abusive situation, while for others it may be difficult. It all depends and still channels back to the level of stress the individual can endure.

Good coping strategy

Anyone who has passed through abuse always faces challenges in coping with the aftermath. Never suppress the feelings of abuse in any way, and always disclose what you are going through to people who are close and supportive to you. When you speak to trusted family members and friends, your stress level will reduce.

When you try to conceal the situation from your family and friends, that is when it affects you even more. Your abuser will have more power to exercise their deadly act; it is like giving them extra bullets for their gun. Other ways of reducing the effects of abuse after the experience is leaving the abusive marriage or relationship. When people quit an abusive relationship or marriage, it gives them the ability to recuperate from their injuries and exhaustion. However, it takes strength and courage to be able to do this.

Many people find it difficult to leave their abusive husband or wife, especially when children are involved. It is a good thing to not want to part with your children, but your own safety and the safety of your children should be your top priority.

If the decision is hard for you to make, think about your life. You deserve a better life. Your children need a happy life. You need to be treated with respect. Ask yourself: What if you or your kids get hurt or killed while in this abusive situation? Stop procrastinating, and take the necessary steps forward to end that relationship or marriage if the abuse continues.

Speak to people that may be able to help you. Involve the authorities, and get the help you need. Most abusers suffer from psychological, emotional, and mental health issues; changing their ways is not as easy as you think. Staying with your abuser does not only endanger you but your children as well. By the time you finally summon the courage and strength to eventually leave your abusive partner, there are things you can do to make you live a meaningful life again.

Understand that abuse is not okay. Our society and everyone around the world frown at it, and it is not something you should accommodate or accept. Be confident and stand up for yourself, and never allow anyone to abusively manipulate you into doing things you would not normally do.

Many of the victims of extreme abuse who delayed when reporting their situation to friends, family, or the authorities never lived to tell their story. Some died by suicide, while others were maimed or killed in cold blood by their abusers. That is why it is important to let people around you know what you are going through, to avoid such a disastrous end.

There are several things you can do to recuperate from your negative experiences. Take time off for a vacation, go to the beach, do yoga, exercise regularly, experience nature more often, make new friends, and do the things that makes you happy. When the above recommendations are followed accordingly, you will soon forget the trauma and stress you went through at the hands of your abuser. Lastly, if the above coping strategies are not playing out to your advantage, you can consult a counsellor or psychologist who can assist you further in overcoming your stress.

Chapter Three
BETRAYAL

ANOTHER KIND OF stressor ravaging people around the world is the stress of betrayal. Most times, it's people very close to us that will betray and backstab us because they know our weak points. They know our secrets, they know everything about us, so they know exactly where to place the knife and stab us. Betrayal stress has ruined lots of lives and relationships around the world. It has ruined long-time friendships, brothers' and sisters' relationships, peers' friendships, and so on. When people confide in you, they trust you, believe in you, and depend on you.

It is not easy for someone to disclose everything about themselves to you, or to open their hearts to you; it takes trust and determination to be able to do that. When people reveal their true identity to you, they see you as their mentor and someone who can put them in the right direction—someone they can wholeheartedly trust. When you disclose people's secrets to others, it is a big betrayal that can destroy their bond with and confidence in you.

It is extremely hard to detect who can betray you. You cannot tell who will betray you by looking at their face. The only sure ways to identify them are through our inner conscience and with time. However, we often do not listen to our inner conscience, due to one distraction or another. Even if we are distracted from identifying the potential betrayers through our feelings, time will definitely expose them.

Those who betray can never permanently conceal their true identity because in one way or the other they will expose themselves to you one day. Betrayals can make some people distrust others, viewing them with suspicion. This can make them shut the doors to their hearts against good people as well. People who have experienced betrayal can start to have low self-esteem, anger, aggression, and a general lack of trust. It could also give them a different meaning to life and can hinder their relationships and associations with people.

The actions of the betrayed person could make them function less in society and could also lead them to negative coping strategies. So, the stress associated with betrayal can be immense and disastrous to many.

Good coping strategy

It is not easy to cope with the stress of being betrayed by the people you trust. We see this play out on social media. People have died by suicide after coming across their naked photos or videos online. Most of these instances are due to betrayal by close friends, boyfriends, girlfriends, or even family members.

Disclosing the secrets of one person to another is a big betrayal. When you find yourself in such a situation, there is no need to always react to it negatively. As the saying goes, "Easier said than done." It's understandable that it's not an easy task to just overlook things like that, but remember, the more you react to it the more harm you do to yourself.

The first thing to do after experiencing betrayal is to forgive the person who has betrayed you; see the betrayal as an eye-opener for you to tread more cautiously with people. When you forgive the person, you are not doing them a favour; rather, you are the beneficiary of that forgiveness. Like the saying goes, "Forgiveness is a gift you give to yourself." When we forgive people who wronged us, we free ourselves from the bondage of getting upset each time we see them.

Forgiving those who have betrayed us does not mean we have to be close to them again; we can set our boundaries and limit the things we do with them. If you happen to live on the same street as someone who has betrayed you, move out of that neighbourhood if possible because the more distance you have from them, the better it will be for you. If you cannot move out from the neighbourhood, distance yourself from them to avoid being hurt again.

Engage yourself in more exercise; go to see live entertainment; read books, go hiking, and experience nature. There is so much more you can do to forget that negative experience of betrayal. This is not to say that there are no faithful friends around—lucky you if you have one! But if you do not have such friends, make God and your soul your most faithful friends.

We all tend to assume that everyone is the same after experiencing betrayal, but we must understand that shutting the doors against everybody because of our experiences with a few people will not be fair to others. Continue to give people that benefit of the doubt; do not just label everyone as the same. When we shut the door of our hearts against everyone, the good people will also not have that chance to come into our lives. Always dissolve the ideas of bad coping strategies because using negative coping strategies like smoking or drinking, as mentioned earlier, can only destroy you; it will not help you in any way.

Chapter Four

DIVORCE

GOING THROUGH THE divorce process is another difficult area of stress that many people go through in life. This is one of the most intense stresses in many communities today. Marriages are being torn apart because of one reason or the other. The most common reason people get divorced is unfaithfulness. Sometimes there are irreconcilable differences, while at other times there is simply a lack of appreciation for one or both spouses. Divorce can cause a lot of damage to people's lives, especially those who do not have the strength to deal with it.

There are many things that can cause divorce—things like lack of appreciation, lack of communication, lack of love, abuse, and dishonesty, to mention a few. When it comes to divorce, it is not what anyone would pray to experience. There are lots of things to put into consideration before deciding to go ahead with divorce, especially those that have children together. People should understand that there is no perfect marriage out there.

Every marriage has its ups and downs. Couples breaking up and going their separate ways can be devastating, which could also lead to a disastrous end. Couples with children should always think about the reaction of their child or children before making that decision of opting out. However, this is not to encourage people to stay in abusive marriages or for them to live with an unfaithful, unloving, or dishonest partner.

The fact is that before you file for a divorce—indeed, before you even have children together—the children should be given consideration because it will have huge negative impact on them. In the absence of abuse, lack of appreciation, extramarital affairs, lack of love and honesty, every other disagreement and occurrence can be sorted out or resolved.

Divorce is like killing the tree you have nurtured to grow, uprooting it after nurturing the tree and then later pulling that same tree down. It takes years to build marriages and only seconds to ruin it. The stress that comes with divorce is outrageous, especially when it is your first time. Experiencing a divorce is different for a variety of people, especially for the one who has put his or her all into making a marriage work.

A partner who cares less about the marriage can feel less pain, but the one who sacrificed their all will find it more difficult to cope. They can still overcome the pain of it, but it will take more time because the stress associated with divorce is too intense and hard to overcome for some people. Coping with such an intense separation could lead to the wrong coping strategies. Therefore, it is particularly important to know the right and best ways to handle it. If people use the wrong coping strategies, it will not only affect their health but also their day-to-day life.

Good coping strategy

Marriage is a good thing that God has ordained for many. Marrying the one we love is supposed to bring happiness, not bitterness. A new marriage is like an empty apartment. When there is nothing in the apartment, we cannot yet enjoy comfort there. But when we start to invest in things to decorate inside the apartment, we will begin to see the beauty and enjoy the comfort. It is the same in marriage. Couples need to contribute to it in equal measure for it to work. Some people get into marriage with expectations, forgetting that they each have a role to play in the marriage to make it work.

The stress associated with divorce is not something anyone wants to experience. To cope with divorce stress, you must be courageous; you have to be optimistic and emotionally strong. Sometimes, when we divorce for the right reasons, we will only stress a little. An example of that is when we divorce for the safety of ourselves and our children. Still, divorce is devastating to all parties involved.

We should learn to understand that without marriage there would have been no divorce, and without divorce there would have been no marriage. When we start to understand the concept of marriage and divorce having a thin line between them, the better we can be able to cope with the stress. The goal of marriage for spouses is to stay together forever and that is why oaths for better for worse are taken between the two to seal the union, but when things start to go wrong that they can't resolve, that is when divorce becomes an option for them. It is not easy for people who grew up in two different backgrounds to live peacefully together. It takes love, faithfulness, understanding, communication, honesty, and constant forgiveness to be able to achieve that goal. If we find ourselves in a divorce situation, we should always understand that something caused it to happen. People do not just get divorced for no reason—there must be some irreconcilable differences that make it happen. Divorce is not always a bad thing, as people may make it seem. Sometimes divorce is for the benefit of the two people whose relationship has dissolved. Sometimes, as soon as they go their separate ways, they both will feel the relief from the stress they had been going through in the relationship.

It is even better for couples who cannot settle their differences to go their separate ways, especially those who have children together. When children see their parents fighting all the time, they will experience adverse psychological effects and damage to their wellbeing, as well as effects in their performance at school. When we do not quit abusive marriages, the effects on our children may come back to haunt us later in life.

Considering the above reasons, it is imperative to file for divorce when the marriage environment is no longer conducive for us and our children. We will still feel the stress, but knowing full well that the decision we have made or about to make is for the benefit of our children and for our peace of mind will give us a little relieve.

Divorce is not always the only way out of every disagreement in marriage. Sometimes understanding that marriage is a commitment, one that requires the cooperation of both parties involved—not a place where one party does all the work—will save us lots of stress.

Divorce is not an easy way out, as some people seem to believe. There are many who use divorce as a means to get out of a relationship and to avoid the hard things that are required to make any relationship work. If our partner doesn't pose a threat to our life and the lives of our children, there are several other resources available to us to help our situation. We can also seek help from therapists to assist us in restoring the peace and harmony we once had in the family.

Chapter Five
PURPOSE AND THE FUTURE

THE REASON WE were created, or the essence of why we exist in the world, is our purpose in life. While our future involves what we plan or assume will likely happen to us later in life, thinking about the future is one of the things stressing many people in our society today. We all think and stress about how our future and the future of our loved ones will look. Each time we are engrossed in these thoughts, it tends to stress us out a lot. Before now, people used to stress less about their future in the world because most of them appreciated what they had and lived below their means. But now there seems to be a spike in the number of people who stress about their future because most of them these days are unsatisfied with what they have.

This spike in number may be due to the changes in the

world today. Some of these changes include, but are not limited to, economic changes, technology changes, relationship, and family changes, among many others.

The above changes always have a huge impact on our day-to-day life. Another thing that can trigger us to stress and worry about the future is the deadly virus, like the pandemic which is ravaging the world right now. Many lives have been lost this pandemic season, and many jobs have been affected too.

There are a lot of people who are living with the stress of uncertainty about their future right now, not knowing what will happen in the next minute, hour, day, week, month or a year from now. The stress of this pandemic is felt more by families who are badly and negatively impacted. Those who have lost their family members to the virus stress way more than those who have not lost any of their family members. These people stress about the future because they believe the future is uncertain for them and their loved ones.

Other things that could stress us about our future is when we have less education, a low-paying job, chronic illness, a lack of physical fitness, and when we are mentally and psychologically unstable. The future is important to every one of us, and that is why most of us worry about it and try to secure it by any means possible. Stress of the future happens to all ages, but it mostly affects individuals who are beyond forty years of age. The more we grow older, the more we become vulnerable to illnesses and prone to decline in physical fitness.

This is the time we start feeling less energetic, and worry and stress about the future affects us more. Many dependent young people do not really worry themselves about the future because most of them are still under the care of their parents. It is their parents who will be thinking about their children's future for them that point in time. Before children get to the legal age to be on their own, their parents must have lectured and prepared them for the future by notifying them about the importance of education and other things that may secure their future for them.

The process of trying to prepare their children for the future stresses many parents out. When most children become teenagers, they believe that they already know all they need to succeed in life. What they fail to realize is that what they think they know in life is just a tip of an iceberg. It requires more knowledge, commitment, dedication, determination, and the grace of God to be able to secure the future. These processes require a lot from us, and that is why it stresses us out when progressing through these phases. Everyone has a different purpose in life, and our purposes cannot be achieved through the same means. The channel your parents, brothers, sisters, and friends went through to achieve their purpose in life is not the same channel you will go through to achieve yours.

We all have different purposes in life; when we try to duplicate other people's channels of achieving their purpose, we become extremely stressed in the process. But when we use the right channel meant for our own purpose in life, the stress will not be as much as when we use other channels not made for our purpose. We all have different purposes in life, and all these purposes require different channels in order to achieve them. When Mr. A tries to achieve Mr. B's purpose, which requires a different channel, Mr. A's results will never work out the same way. That is why many people in the world today lose track of their true purpose in life and will stress even more to secure their future with the wrong purpose in their minds.

Your true purpose in life is the most important thing you should take note of because if you miss your true purpose in life there is nothing you will do that will make you happy. It is only when you are on track with your true purpose in life that you will have that inner peace of fulfillment.

Good coping strategy

Stressing over the future happens to almost every individual in the world. It is natural for us to stress over our future because we literally do not know what tomorrow may bring. One thing we should understand is that we all have different futures and different purposes in life. All purpose in life requires different channels in achieving them; just because your friends or relatives achieved their true purpose and secured their future through certain channels does not mean that the same channels will work for you.

Many people in the world today are in prison, or get themselves in one sort of trouble or the other, just because they try using the same channel as their friends or relatives to achieve their purpose to secure their future. We all have different questions when it comes to our purpose in life, and it requires different answers to those questions. That is why even if we teach other people how to achieve their purpose in life or secure their future, most of them will still fail in the process because the answers to their questions are different from ours.

We know that our future is important, and just as our future is important to us, our physical, mental, and psychological wellbeing are important as well. We should not stress carelessly about our future to the extent where it will start affecting our physical, mental, and psychological wellbeing. Let us always learn to live in the present and plan wisely towards the future without stressing too much about it. The world is full of challenges and uncertainties; these challenges and uncertainties were already here on earth before we were even born, so stressing and worrying about them will do us more harm than good.

It's not advisable to always stress ourselves about the future, but if you are bent on securing your future at all cost, you should make sure the following are already in place in your life: God's presence, a good education, a professional trade or training and recognizing the things you are good at. These skills will allow you to effectively plan for your future; however, it does not guarantee a secure future. The only one who can guarantee a secure future is God; beyond that, you must know your purpose in life. When you know your purpose in life, you will enjoy every bit of the journey to the future.

Most times it is through knowing God and doing his will that you can figure out your life purpose. Meeting with God one-on-one and adhering to his instructions grants us the ability to achieve our purpose in life. Other things you could do to cope with the stress of the future is to engage yourself in exercise and yoga, and to socialize. When we socialize with people, do yoga, and exercise our body, we relax our muscles, ease our tension, and give ourselves the ability to perform mindful meditation, which will in turn reduce our stress.

If we don't do these things, we tend to get angrier over

our situation, and when we are angry it affects our cognitive ability to make the right and important decisions of our lives. Apart from getting involved with exercise, yoga, and socializing, you could also seek the services of a professional counselor who can walk you through stress-relief programs to help you better cope with the stress of the future.

Additionally, always have it in mind that in the absence of God's presence in your life, it will not be easy to know your purpose in life. And in order to secure your future, you need to know your purpose. When you know your purpose, most of the things required to secure your future will automatically fall into place and allow you to fulfill that purpose. The word of God declares through the holy bible about our purpose in life:

Psalm 33:11: But the plans of the LORD stand firm forever, the purposes of his heart through all generations.

Romans 8:28: And we know that for those who love God, all things work together for good, for those who are called according to his purpose.

Jeremiah 1:5: Before I formed you in the womb, I knew you, and before you were born, I consecrated you; I appointed you a prophet to the nations.

Another thing is that we can strive to know our purpose in life, but we do not have to stress and worry about it. As it says in Matthew 6:34: Take therefore no thought for morrow; for the morrow shall take thought for the things of itself. Sufficient unto the day is the evil thereof.

This means that we should not worry too much about the things of tomorrow or the future, and that the future will take care of itself—and that the trouble for today is already enough for us.

Chapter Six
NATURAL DISASTER

NATURAL DISASTER HAS placed many people in devastating situations and has caused several others life-altering experiences. Every year around the world, millions of people go through stress from natural disasters. Natural disasters could include earthquakes, floods, tsunamis, fires, tornadoes, explosions, and many more. Any time a natural disaster occurs in any nation, loss of lives, properties, and other valuables are negatively impacted.

People could lose their entire families, houses, valuables, or even their entire communities to natural disaster. When people experience these things, they go through extreme stress, and when they go through stress they will began to act inappropriately. The negative impact of stress can begin to affect their everyday life. Natural disaster is what people pray not to ever experience, and when it does happen people are at risk of both emotional and physical health challenges. After every natural disaster, people affected go through stress; some may recover, and others may not. However, it depends on the level of damages the disaster has caused the individuals or persons and how well they can handle stress.

The people who experience the worst impact of natural disasters are those who have lost their entire family members and properties. To these people life is worthless; to them there is nothing go live for, and to them nature is ruthless. It only takes the grace of God for them to recover from their loss. Just imagine waking up one morning, afternoon, or night and to find out that all your family members and properties are gone. Picture how you will feel knowing full well there is nothing to hold on to nor a place to go.

The stress associated with some natural disasters are too extreme for some people to endure. Coping with such losses are too challenging for many people; they cannot simply push this loss aside and just move on. It requires lots of treatments, therapy, and counselling before they can recover from the shock of losing everything.

Good coping strategy

Coping with the tragedy of natural disaster is not easy, but there are strategies we can use to manage it. These strategies might work for some people and might not work for others; it all depends on the level of damage the natural disaster has caused. Most natural disasters do not give signs before they strike; it is a sudden occurrence caused by nature. Natural disaster can happen anywhere around the world, but there are known specific countries or areas in the world that are more vulnerable.

When natural disaster occurs in any country, people tend to lose most of their possessions and things that may continue to affect them in their daily lives. It is understandable that it is not easy to forget all of the damages a natural disaster may have caused you or those around you. The first thing that should cheer you up after natural disaster is the fact that you are still alive. Think about the people who lost their lives in the tragedy; think about young children whose parents lost their lives and made them orphans; think about those that are disfigured by the disaster and think about those who lost their properties, their most valuable things—including their lives.

When we think about these scenarios mentioned above, we should have reasons to glorify God for giving us another chance to live. You should not allow the stress of natural disaster take total control of your physical and mental well-being; you are still the one in the driver's seat of your life. Remember that, aside from God, you are still in charge of your life, and whatever decisions you make can have a huge impact on what your life will become.

If you still have family members and friends left, spend more time with them. When you are around your good friends or family members, your stress level tends to reduce drastically. If you lost all your family members and friends in the disasters, there are still other resources you could use to help reduce your stress. You could attend counselling sessions; you could see a psychologist; you could see therapists and other medical experts or agencies who could help in one way or the other to better your situation.

All the things you should be doing are those that can bring solutions and not additional problems. Another thing you could do is to move far away from reminders of the disaster. When you limit your exposure to these reminders, you are not likely to have too many reflections about the disastrous event. Try to engage in positive things that could lighten up your spirit rather than just remaining there and sobbing over the tragedy. Consider the tragedy as the past and put everything concerning it in the past. Talk about it only when you need to and not every minute of the day; do not rush things; do things step by step.

Do not allow anyone to push you to do things you are not mentally ready for; you should do those things whenever it suits you. And remember that it is all about you and not those people who may be trying to influence your decisions. They are not the ones directly involved in the mess; that is why you do not have to agree to everything they say. You should avoid any forms of bad coping strategies, like excessive smoking, drinking, or drug use. If you do these things, you will later regret doing them because drug use will not only restrict you from reaching your full potential in life, it could also destroy your life.

Chapter Seven

COPYING OTHERS

COPYING THE LIFESTYLE of other people is another stress many individuals go through. When you start to copy people, you are telling yourself that you are not doing enough in life. It is like you do not appreciate what you have and that you are ungrateful to God. You will begin to have low self-esteem and negative thoughts towards yourself. Remember, "all that glitters is not gold." When you see people living a certain lifestyle, most especially when they are living life above their means, ask yourself: Does that person earn more than they could spend? Some people you see popping bottles in the club do not really have money—most of them are trying to impress others and make them believe that they are living a fulfilling life, but in reality, they go home and soak their pillows with tears.

Most of these people showing off on social media—taking pictures with expensive cars, houses, and wearing the latest designer outfits—could be the highest debtor around. Living a fake life is one of the worst decisions anyone can make. Most of the things you see on social media are not true; they are just displays put on by people trying to paint themselves as something they are not. Many marriages, relationships, and friendships that took years to build have been destroyed by fake lifestyles.

Faking someone else's lifestyle will not only stress you out, it could also negatively affect your wellbeing and change it forever. Most of the people copying the lifestyle of others face anxiety on a daily basis; hearing their phone beep or ring always create panic in their minds, making them restless. Some of the things that come to their minds are: Who is that person messaging me? Have they found out my true identity? What have they found out? Who is monitoring me? I hope nobody finds out! These are the things that will be circulating in the hearts of those copying others, which also makes them restless and uncomfortable.

There is a popular quote stated in one of this book's chapters, which says, "The greatest prison anyone can live in is the fear of what others think of them." If you take a closer look at this quote, you will realize that it's actually true because when you are constantly worried about what other people think of you, it means you are living in their prison.

Good coping strategy

Living a fake life is no longer new in our society. Some people will never feel good about themselves until they lie to impress others. When people live a fake life, they believe that they are doing the right thing, but unknown to them they are literally hurting themselves. Many individuals have done what they would not have normally done in the process of impressing others.

Anytime we copy the lifestyle of other people, we are being ungrateful to God. There is stress associated with not being satisfied with what we have. When people believe that they do not have as much as others, they stress over it. Many people have got into big trouble in the process of trying to live the lifestyle of other people. We should live our lives the best way we can and be content with what we have.

Most times, people that we are trying to copy don't even have half of the things we are blessed with or have internally, but still we are so carried away with their physical looks and the things they are doing. Many such people are living in debt and on their credit cards, and sometimes those things we see them with are borrowed from friends or family members. When we appreciate what we have and are content, we do not have to stress over anything like that.

Always keep cool with things in life and live a life of contentment. Do things according to your strength, and never allow social media or any other platform to negatively influence your way of life. Social media has caused lots of damage to marriages, relationships, and friendships. Don't copy what you see on social media because most of what you see there is untrue.

Never live above your means, and live within your budget. Surround yourself with responsible people who do not show off or try to impress others with what is not even their own. Avoid people living fake lifestyles; distance yourself from them so that you can concentrate on the most important things in life. People living fake lives are distractions to others because they paint themselves as what they are not, and they make others regret who they are. Turn a blind eye to the things they do; see them as impostors, and never believe anything they say to you. Appreciate what you have, believe in yourself, and do things within your financial capacity.

Chapter Eight
UNEMPLOYMENT

JOBLESSNESS IS ANOTHER trigger that can cause stress in people's lives. When one's income stops coming in from its source, it can create a whole lot of chaos in the family. Joblessness does not only affect the person—it affects their entire family. Imagine going to work one day and getting laid off or fired. This could be a life-changing scenario that can have huge negative impact on you if it is not well handled.

This is the point where people would start stressing over their mortgages, children's education, car loans, and other loans that have been taken from the banks or lenders. When somebody is idle and doing nothing, that is when they start thinking different kinds of negative things that could worsen their situation. Idle men can easily give in to temptations that come their way. But keeping themselves busy will make them concentrate on the positive things of life.

People handle joblessness differently. To some, it's no big deal—when they lose their employment, they may say, "Oh well, it was just a job." To others, it will look as if their whole life has ended due to all the financial obligations and commitments they have already made. It all depends on the individual, and that is why it is imperative to understand how much stress we can take, and to always prepare for uncertainties.

It is not easy to figure out our stress levels individually, but it is something that is possible and important to know. If our stress level can be recognized, it will be possible to keep it from escalating to an uncontrollable level. When we lose our jobs and have bills piling up, we experience a stressful phase of life.

Good coping strategy

There are different phases of life on earth: we have the good ones, the tough ones, and the bad ones. The earlier we understand these phases of life, the better for us to cope with them. This life is full of ups and downs, and we should not believe that things will always be smooth for us. One minute things can be good and fine, and the other minute things can change for the worse. We should always have this at the back of our minds so that when hard times strike, we will be able to handle it.

If you look at most people who have experienced intense stress, they are those who only believe that this life is only one way and that things will always be good.

Even God himself did not promise us freedom from trouble in the world; the only thing he assured us is that he will *overcome* the troubles in the world. When he said he will overcome the world, he simply meant that he will give us the *ability* to overcome troubles—and in that verse he wasn't talking to unbelievers, he was in fact talking to those that believed in him. What does he mean by the ability he promised us to overcome troubles? He means he will give us the strength to handle troubles when they strike.

This reference to the bible indicates some clarity that life cannot always be smooth as many people may think; we must experience good times, tough times, and bad times. The earlier we adapt ourselves to these changes in life, the better for us to cope with them. When we do not have a job, it is not the end of the world because when one door closes, another one opens. We must always be optimistic that things will always get better, no matter the situation.

So, losing our jobs is not a life sentence that we should grieve and sob over for a long time. We should see it as an opportunity to explore the different phases of life, which also allows us to gain more experience in life. As it is often said: If we haven't yet seen something in our lives, it simply means we haven't yet arrived at the destination. Remember too that experience is our best teacher.

Chapter Nine

HARASSMENT

HARASSMENT HAPPENS EVERY day around the world, and in many different settings. However, workplace harassment is the first kind that we will elaborate on in this chapter. This is another stressor many employees experience from their colleagues or employers in many workplaces. Studies have shown that there is a high percentage of women who are constantly harassed in their workplaces. Women have always experienced harassment, especially the sexual nature of it, in their places of work.

This is not to say that men do not experience sexual harassment—they do indeed—but women are more vulnerable to it. To be sexually harassed in a workplace or anywhere outside work is another stressor that has affected and still affecting many individuals today. The scariest part of sexual harassment is when one encounters it with a total stranger. Imagine being sexually harassed by a stranger on your way to work. That experience will trigger a whole lot of trauma in your life.

Sexual harassment in Western countries are well handled by law enforcement officers because they have all the necessary interviewing, interrogative, and investigative skills to figure out how the offence may have occurred. However, it could take months, years, or even decades to conclude investigations to bring the culprits to justice. Being able to treat cases of this nature and sentencing perpetrators is most important to their victims. Victims might not immediately recover after the attack, but penalizing perpetrators of that evil act can have a huge positive impact on the victim's recovery process.

In some parts of the world, such as in some Third World countries, these crimes are not taken seriously, or perhaps they lack the skill and equipment to investigate such cases. Just imagine been continually harassed in your workplace while nothing is been done to stop it or to protect the victims. Millions of people in Third World countries face various kinds of harassment in their workplaces and neighbourhoods each day, without adequate police protection or investigations into these crimes.

Imagine the level of stress these people are going through at the hands of their attackers. The stress of being a victim of harassment of any nature is one thing, and the stress of not being protected from perpetrators is still another. Human beings are created differently. There are people who may not want to report issues of harassment in their workplaces, neighbourhoods, or other public places because of their low self-esteem, fear of losing their job, or fear of being killed. That is why it is important to report to the authorities when we know anyone that is going through harassment.

If we refuse to step in, the situation may get worse and may lead the person involved into depression, which could eventually make them attempt suicide or use the wrong coping strategies. Helping somebody going through harassment stress is like saving their life. Harassment stress is not something we can endure or deal with alone; we need the help of other people or the authorities to be able to handle it.

Some people are slow to respond to things happening to them due to fear of being laughed at or mocked. That is why it takes some of them several years or even decades to be able to speak up. We cannot completely absorb the effects of harassment by ourselves, alone; when we try to do that, we are destroying ourselves, which will directly affect us and prevent us from reaching our full potential in life. When we accept the things we are not supposed to accept, it pulls us back and limits us from achieving greater things.

Good coping strategy

It's not easy to cope with harassment stress, especially when it involves total strangers. The experience may change the way we see others by making us assume everyone is the same. It may stop us from trusting people, including those close to us. Harassment comes with stress that can limit our progress in whatever we do, so we should not take it lightly. The first thing we should do is to take notes of the incidents from the moment it happened, and describe *how* it happened, by using the four W's: Who, what, where, and when: *who* caused the incident; *what* was the nature of the incident; *where* the incident happened, and *when*. We should also make note of *how* the incident happened.

This information can assist in investigations when things eventually escalate. Another thing you should do is to talk about the incident, with somebody close to you—someone you trust to have a high level of integrity. In doing so, you create potential witnesses who could help you testify against the perpetrator. Harassers are quick to deny the things they have done without a blink of an eye because they know they can get in big trouble.

That is why it is imperative to keep track of the whole incident. Sometimes we can easily forget certain things, such as the dates they happened, where they happened, the time they happened, and the people involved. But with our notes we can easily reflect on these things. When we have this information to back our claims, it reduces our stress level, but when we have no information or evidence to back our claims, it aggravates our stress level.

You can help yourself by engaging in things you enjoy doing; take care of yourself in the best possible ways. Treat yourself to nice things that will always give you joy; this will help lift your spirits should you feel defeated or down. Always see yourself as a winner and not a loser. Exercise often, and keep your head up; eat healthy foods to energize your body because you need that strength to fight the battle ahead of you. Giving up should never be an option for you, and if at any point you feel like giving up, seek professional assistance.

Chapter Ten
INCREASE IN FINANCIAL OBLIGATIONS

INCREASING OUR FINANCIAL obligations can aggravate our stress to a higher level when not done at the appropriate time. Anxiety and depression are the two most common reactions to financial stress, and they can lead us to many health problems. Some people do not wait till they are ready to do certain things in life before doing them. There is time for everything, most especially around our finances. Do not say that your friend did it, so you are going to do it too. That is not the way it works. You should always be ready before engaging yourself in activities that create more financial obligations.

There are people who have drowned in debt just

because they did not wait for the appropriate time to increase their financial obligations. Before you increase your financial obligations, there are things you need to keep in mind. You will need to make accurate calculations of your earnings. For example, think about your job. Is it a full-time job? Do some research on the company you work for and try to learn about the performance of the company. If a layoff should occur right now, will you be affected? These are some of the things you should figure out first before increasing your financial obligations.

Another thing to keep in mind is your medical status. Are you physically fit to continue working and earning the same amount in the next decade? If you are the type that does two jobs, ask yourself if you would be able to continue working the two jobs for a long time.

Some people do not think about these things before increasing their financial obligations. That is why, when things go wrong, it will be a surprise to them and eventually land them in a state of extreme stress. When you put the above scenarios into consideration before engaging yourself in more financial obligations, it will be difficult for you to get stressed out over it should anything happen to your job. In addition, some of these people are pushed into this financial stress by those close to them—their partners, friends, or even family members.

That is why you should surround yourself with people who will add good value to your life and not those who will add stress to it. Increasing your financial obligations without proper planning could place you in extremely stressful conditions. When you find yourself in those conditions, you may become vulnerable to bad coping strategies.

Good coping strategy

To comfortably increase your financial obligations, make sure certain things are in place. First, you must make calculations of the streams of income you have, such as all the money coming in and going out. You need to evaluate your financial status and prepare for the worst-case scenario should any of your income channels shuts down or stop.

There are ups and down in this life, and most things are not permanent. Before increasing your financial obligations, you should always have an open mind to the possibility of things changing, and prepare yourself for such changes. If you do not prepare yourself against the worst-case scenarios, that is when the stress associated with increasing your financial obligations will hit you extremely hard.

When you prepare yourself against the uncertainties of life, there is a possibility that you will not even feel the negative impact of stress. Additionally, you should always do things within your power, things you know you can easily deal with no matter your financial circumstances. Living above your means or doing things outside the capacity of your financial strength is not worth it.

Like the saying goes, "Sew your coat according to your size." When you live within your financial capacity, you stress less over things that have to do with finances. Always remember that things easily fade away. That thing you are so excited about today may become useless tomorrow—always remember that.

When the prices of desired items are high and above your financial capability, wait for their prices to drop before buying them. Also, there are people who buy things they do not really need just because they are addicted to shopping. Try to take control of your spending habits by figuring out the things you need and those you do not need. If possible, create other potential streams of income when possible, and use them as backups in case your current one stops.

Another thing you could do is talk about your financial situation to the people you trust. This could be your family members or friends—somebody you know will not use your financial situation against you or mock you; bear in mind that some people are quick to judge others. If your friends are the sympathetic type, they might come up with brilliant ideas on how you can get your finances under control. The surest ways of coping with our financial stress is by taking control of our finances, understanding the causes of our financial stressors, building streams of income, increasing our financial needs at the appropriate time, living within our budgets, and adjusting ourselves to the lifestyles we know we can easily maintain.

Chapter Eleven
CHRONIC ILLNESS OR INJURY

ANOTHER STRESSOR THAT could have a huge negative impact on people is when they have chronic illness or injury. Remember, there are ups and downs in life, in which there are uncertainties that cannot be controlled. No one knows what is going to happen the next second, next minute, next hour or next day. Imagine waking up in the morning and feeling really sick with chronic illness, or going to work and sustaining a catastrophic injury.

When people encounter the above examples, they always go through extreme stress. Chronic illnesses and injuries are things that happen suddenly to people, and it is not what they expect to happen to them. And when it does happen, it can have huge negative impact on their wellbeing and life in general. That negative impact changes into stress over time, and that could lead to other devastating issues.

Having chronic illness or injury can get worse, especially when you do not have good family members and friends around you, or if you do not have adequate finances to take care of yourself. It could be even more devastating and stressful when you don't get the help you really need on time, but when you do get the help you need and on time, there is possibility to recover fast from your illness or injury. When people are healthy, without any illness or injury, they tend to be independent and do practically everything for themselves.

But when they become immobile and their physical abilities are restricted, that is where the challenges are and when they start to have problems in their life, which will allow stress to kick in. And when they start having stress, they become miserable in their day-to-day life, which could possibly affect people around them if not properly taken care of.

Good coping strategy

Chronic illness or injury is not what anyone would wish to have or experience in life; however if it does happen, it should not be the end of our lives or seen as a life sentence. Chronic illnesses or injuries can be managed when we get the appropriate help and assistance we need. The first thing you can do when you have either one of the above conditions is to feed your soul with thoughts of things getting better, and not giving up on yourself, and this is the time you need to think positively.

When you are positive about your predicament, things

will improve for you, but when you give up on yourself and always think negatively, it could worsen things for you. Try to understand your illness or injury to the best of your ability, and adhere to your healthcare professional's advice and instructions. Do not allow things you know will make you unhappy as well as those that may be detrimental to your health.

Get in the habit of taking your medications, according to your doctor's instructions—and on time, too. Go to places and meet people who will bring out the best in you, not those who will add to your problems. Do not be in denial of your situation because trying to deny that you are sick or have an injury will only make your situation worse. Accept your problems the way they are. When you accept them, that gives you total control of your situation as well as the solution to those problems. It is only when you accept your problem that solutions to them will start to manifest.

Do not worry if your first strategy does not work; keep trying other good coping strategies till they work out for you. Giving up shouldn't be an option for you because if you give up on yourself, your whole body will start to give up on you, so don't give your body the opportunity to give up on you. Another thing you should do is to continue taking care of yourself the way you used to because if you do not take care of yourself, your overall health condition may become weaker and weaker.

Try to engage with any exercises that are within your restrictions; do not become inactive. When you exercise regularly, your body becomes active and lighter. In addition, you should be grateful to God in whatever situation you find yourself; always remember too that there are people out there who may be facing worse situations than the one you have. The bible teaches that in all situations, we should always give thanks to our creator.

Chapter Twelve
GETTING MARRIED

GETTING MARRIED IS the dream of every man and woman; however, going through the preparation process can be stressful to the couple. Once the date of wedding is fixed or announced by the couple, that is the day they start stressing out over the preparations. Many people have gone through pre-wedding stress in one way or the other. There are lots of things to be done when planning a wedding, and when these things are not put in place before the wedding day, they tend to stress the couples out.

Those who have the money to hire a wedding planner do not have to stress as much; they will still be stressed a little, but not as much as those doing the preparations themselves. The most stressful part of the wedding is when all the arrangements made did not come out the way they were planned—especially if the couple does not have enough finances to cover it and has to take out a loan for the wedding. Other stressful things can happen: What if the photographer doesn't show up or doesn't properly capture important parts of the ceremony? Perhaps the cake is not ready on time, the groomsmen and bridesmaids are not all at the wedding venue, or the wedding dress is not ready—or, even worse, the wedding dress or suit doesn't fit properly. Perhaps the groom or bride are delayed on their way to the wedding venue. These and many other things can bring great stress to a wedding.

The above examples could stress out partners who are planning to get married. Other things that could stress couples out are members of both families, especially when they are not in agreement with each other. Things like lack of parental approval to get married, or arguments over how the wedding should be done. These things could cause lots of tension and chaos between couples when taking care of their preparations. Weather is another factor that could stress couples out; this is something that is totally out of your control.

There are so many other things that could happen to you when you are under pre-wedding stress. You might start to lose interest in sex; stress might reduce your appetite for food, or it might cause you headache and sleeplessness, among other things. If these stressors are not effectively managed, it could lead to fights and disagreements between couples—and if care is not taken the couple might end up breaking up. So, it's important to prepare ourselves physically, mentally, and psychologically before engaging ourselves in wedding preparations.

Good coping strategy

Getting married should be a thing of joy and happiness, an event that creates good memories—not the other way around. Stressing over things that will bring happiness to our lives is not a good start. Before the wedding, you should concentrate on the things you can control, not those beyond your control; doing so will reduce your stress. For example, the weather is not something you can control; instead of stressing over weather, worrying that it might rain or snow, you should channel your energy towards the things under your control.

You should set out time to work on your wedding plans and not sink your thoughts, every minute of the day, into planning your wedding. For example, you can plan to think about your wedding for three hours a day, two to three times a week (depending on the amount of time you have left until the big day). Use your three hours on whatever days you choose to work on your planning. Do not use all your free time planning your wedding; do other things you enjoy too; this will make you happy during the planning process as well.

We cannot continue to stress ourselves day after day just because we are getting married. We should limit ourselves from some things like texts and phone calls. When some texts or calls comes in, we should take our time to answer them so that we will not make any mistakes on our orders in the process. Most times, when we hastily respond to sensitive things like wedding preparation messages or calls from people, we tend to make mistakes; that is why it is important to take our time before responding to them.

When we do take our time, it allows us to seek different opinions before making our final decisions. We should take time to meditate to help us see things from different perspectives, which will also give us more clarity of the things we are about to do. If you are aspiring to get married, you should learn to prepare financially for life after the marriage, not spending all you have in preparation for the marriage.

There are cases of separations and divorces after months, weeks, or even days after marriage due to financial issues. Your priority should be the life you will live after getting married, not sinking yourself in debt to please other people at your wedding. This is not to say that holding an expensive or luxury wedding is not good, but doing it when we are capable will save us lots of stress after the big day.

Chapter Thirteen
MOVING TO A NEW HOME

BUYING AND MOVING into a new home is the dream of every family, but there are lots of stressors associated with it as well. The process of moving is not as easy as some people may think, especially when we do not have good friends or family members around that can help us in the process. Even if we pay movers to help us with our properties, there are still lots of things to do after moving. Movers have limits to what they can help you with; they cannot help us arrange our properties after moving them. We will have to do all our property arrangements ourselves with the help of friends or family members.

In the event of not having reliable friends or family members, we will feel the pressure and stress even more. There are many cases where people fall sick after moving from their old home to a new one. Some people fall sick after moving because they could not absorb the stress associated with moving. After we have moved, it does not end there: we will have to arrange everything all over again, and this could take an exceptionally long time.

It could take months or even years to arrange your belongings the way you really want them or to the exact places you really want them to be. Arranging light things is okay to do, but arranging the heavy pieces, like huge furniture or electronics, is a big challenge. Moving these heavy belongings stresses people out; even after arranging all of our belongings in our homes, we can still wake up one morning and decide to rearrange them again, which will require the assistance of friends or family members.

Making decisions about where each property will go also stresses people out. Imagine getting help from a friend or family member to move some heavy furniture from one spot to another and the next day you find that the pieces of furniture in those new spots do not look good there. And the people or persons who had helped you moved the pieces of furniture has already left. The thoughts of moving them from their current spots to another is what drains people and stresses them out.

Maybe we called for help from the initial helpers and they told us they would not be able to come back to assist us anymore. Their refusal to assist us again will definitely stress us out.

Good coping strategy

Moving to new home can be incredibly stressful to most people. While it is joyful to buy a new home and move into it, when we do not get the help that we need we become stressed out. The first and foremost thing we should understand is that stress is normal when moving from one place to another. Acknowledging that fact will not only reduce our stress, but it will also strengthen us during the moving process.

When we anticipate things before they come our way, there won't be any surprises when they eventually come because we already know what to expect. Another thing you can do is to stay organized. When we organize ourselves before the moving day, it gives us total control over the whole process because we already arranged and packed our things. It also allows us to know where our most prized valuables are, as well as all our fragile stuff.

We do not have to be in a hurry when moving; it should be on a step-by-step basis. Do not leave everything till the last minute; preplan your moving time. When you preplan, it will make things easier for you on moving day. We should not assume we will finish moving at a certain time because timing yourself will give you tension that could aggravate your stress level.

Take it easy when moving; too much rushing may even make you destroy your fragile valuables or even make you misplace your important documents or other valuables, which will throw you into more stress. Give yourself enough time to avoid rushing because rushing things can disorganize your thinking. Some people like to do things at the last minute, and when they do that, they place themselves in a tight corner which will eventually make them rush things during moving. The process of rushing to get things done faster can aggravate your stress level.

When your moving date is approaching, you should try to get enough sleep as much as you can because when we sleep and get enough rest, moving will be much easier for us. Getting enough rest will energize us and prepare us for moving day, but if we do not get enough rest, we will become too tired to function properly on that day.

Furthermore, you can hire good professional movers who can help you with the fragile, bulky and larger items in your home, like washing machines, couches, televisions, bed sets, dressers, as well as other huge pieces that you know you cannot carry alone. Not all movers have the good heart to assist you wholeheartedly with these huge items. There have been cases where some movers will agree to move all your heavy and bulky items, and then somewhere along the line, they will only end up moving only few of them and they will disappear. So, it is important to use known professional movers that have an office, professionals you will be able to trace and not those people you only find online, and don't pay in full until all your properties are moved to the agreed location.

Before the moving date, try to confirm the location of their office and confirm your booking in person, and not over the phone; this will help you to avoid further stress in case the movers do not show up. In addition, there are some moving professionals who collects people's money through online email transfer and end up not showing up. That is why it is important to go to their office to confirm their location before making any form of payment.

When we do not take these precautions, we are bound to fall victim to the fraudsters among these movers. Falling prey to such fraudulent companies will increase our stress level during our moving process. If the moving cost does not fit in your budget, you can ask for help from good, reliable, and trusted family members or friends. Use people you know can voluntarily help you move safely; if you do not have any family members or friends around you, then you can seek the assistance of a trusted professional movers.

Chapter Fourteen
TAKING CARE OF A SICK FAMILY MEMBER

TAKING CARE OF a sick family member can be devastating and stressful. When a family member is sick, the only options available to other family members are to either take care of them or abandon them. Most people would prefer to care for their family member rather than abandoning them to their faith. That is why building a good relationship with each other is very important. When there is good relationship between one another, there is possibility of helping each other out at the time of need.

Every good man or woman would not abandon their family member for any reason. Although, in some cases, some family members deserve to be abandoned; it all depends on what has transpired between the family member who is volunteering to help and the other family member who needs the help. When you assist any family member and they refuse to appreciate what you have done for them, this can sometimes turn off the feelings you have for them. However, learn to always do things for people without expecting appreciation from them; that way, their reactions will not stress you out, even if they don't appreciate what you've done for them.

You should always assist whoever needs your help, whether it's family members, friends or those you don't even know. Always remember that anyone that loves you, cares about you, and treats you right is your family; it's not always by blood. This is not to say that some family members would not still abandon one another. There are some family members who, no matter what you do for them, will still find an excuse not to render you help at the point of need.

The most difficult part of engaging oneself in taking care of a sick loved one is when they cannot do anything for themselves at all. Family members in such critical condition need more help than ever because they practically depend on you for everything. Even if they depend on you to do everything for them, it is always imperative to help them out, especially when they are ill.

Helping a sick family member is not an easy task. It takes love, courage, tolerance, understanding and patience, and it can be incredibly stressful. When we see people taking care of their loved ones, we should always try to commend their efforts and appreciate what they are doing.

When we do this, we are encouraging them as well as giving them strength during their difficult and stressful times.

Caring for a sick family member can restrict you from many important things in your own life. Some of the restrictions include limited socializing with other people close to you, having fewer years of formal education, and obstacles to many other things that will move your life forward. When something is restricting us from doing the things that make us happy, we are bound to stress out over it.

There are other difficulties that we may go through while taking care of our loved ones. We will began to lose interest in the things we used to enjoy doing; we will began to have sleepless nights; we may start having headaches and migraines; we may get easily irritated and upset over little things; our finances will began to plunge, which will make our stress level skyrocket.

Good coping strategy

The first thing that should come to our minds when we are requested or mandated to take care of our loved ones is placing ourselves in their shoes. When we place ourselves in their shoes, we realize we would ask them for a similar favour if the case was the other way round. Realizing that this illness could have happened to anyone will reduce the stress we will have to go through when caring for them.

When we are caring for a sick family member, we easily forget about our own health and our life. A whole lot can go wrong when we do not plan properly before taking care of our loved ones. Illnesses don't give notice before they strike, and most times we don't really have enough time to plan—but we can still set up some things for the people around us to help us with. When we are hit with the responsibility of caring for people we love, sometimes we may have some sympathetic people around us, like friends who may render us helping hands. This is not something that happens all the time, but in some cases a few people may want to help us out.

People who wish to help may do things like running errands, doing laundry, or even buying groceries for us. When they volunteer to render us help, no matter how little, we should not reject it—in fact, we should accommodate every possible form of help we can get. Another thing is that you should not feel you are not doing enough for the sick person and should acknowledge that you are doing your absolute best to help better their situation. You should get as much rest as you can because when you get enough rest, you will feel stronger and have enough energy to care for the sick one, so caring for yourself is very important too.

Find time to exercise your body because when you do exercises, it clears your mind and brings enough oxygen to your brain, which will make you function properly when helping the sick family member. That way, you will not feel irritated or get angry at things that do not even warrant it. While caring for a loved one, never, never forget your own health because many are quick to forget about themselves and then get sick afterwards. Make sure you eat healthy foods, drink lots of water, and take care of yourself; find time to do things that make you happy.

If at any time things are not improving for your sick family member, and your own life is gradually taking a wrong turn for spending too much time with them, or if your own health is affected and at risk, you can always seek professional assistance by moving the family member to a long-term care home where you can visit them regularly. Also, you can use other alternatives available to you. For example, if you feel it won't be fair for them to go to long-term care home, you can equally seek the services of personal support workers or long-term caregivers who could come into your home to care for the sick family member.

Chapter Fifteen
WORKING UNDER DANGEROUS CONDITIONS

TO HAVE A job is one thing, but to have one that keeps us working under dangerous conditions is another. When people work under dangerous conditions, there is always fear of the unknown, along with chaos and sadness in those people's minds whenever they go to work. Some people might even develop post-traumatic stress disorder (PTSD) during their careers. Imagine going to work every day with the knowledge that hazards are all around where you are working.

Compared to the rest of the world, Western countries have the safest environments in which to work. Their govern-ments always put in place precautions and policies to make sure everyone is safe in every workplace. As well, they set up monitoring bodies or agencies to make sure these rules are properly followed; there are penalties companies can face when they breach or violate the rules. In most Third World countries, these safety rules are not followed by many companies, even when the government makes it mandatory.

Bribery and corruption have taken over the leadership of most Third World countries. This is not to say that Westerners do not face the fear or stress of working in dangerous conditions, but they have better chances of less stress in their workplaces. Let us go back to the stress associated with working in dangerous conditions. When we work in dangerous conditions, we fear injuries, death, and the unknown. We may start to have reflections in the dream when we are asleep, and these reflections can start to drain us and make us unhappy.

We could start to develop PTSD, and when we start to have that we will start to lose concentration and focus at work. And when we lose concentration and focus at work, this could lead us to a stressful and disastrous end. This time, people will not only be endangering themselves, but also people in that work environment. Another scenario we could use is this pandemic season of the spread of coronavirus also known as COVID-19; exposure to this virus is an example of working in dangerous conditions.

In some countries, thousands of lives have been lost to this virus, and millions of cases are still pending around the globe. Our doctors, nurses, personal support workers, and many other healthcare professionals risk their lives every day to care for patients who may have the virus or those who may have been exposed to it. Imagine the stress they go through each day for fear of contacting the virus.

Many healthcare workers have equally lost their lives in the line of duty while trying to save others. They all go through stress knowing the kind of virus they are exposed to; this is especially difficult for those healthcare workers who have young children at home. The stress associated with the fear of getting infected is what drains healthcare professionals most—not the actual virus. There are other occupations where people are exposed to dangerous hazards, like malfunctioning equipment or slippery floors. Often, people are not provided with proper safety gears, sometimes improper labelling of safety hazards, improperly illustrated safety rules, and untagged equipment that is unsafe to use.

The above examples do not only physically expose us to danger, they also emotionally affect our wellbeing. The emotional and physical effects of stress include: reduced interest in sex; breathing heavily; loss of appetite; headaches; fatigue; excessive sweating; tension in your muscles; and pains in your body.

Good coping strategy

When we work under dangerous conditions, we are always scared and restless. That fear and restlessness can easily trigger our moods and can negatively impact our performance and productivity. The initial thing you can do is to understand the things that are causing you stress and to voice your concerns to your employer of those things making you feel unsafe in that environment. In most countries, workers have the right to refuse unsafe work, so anytime you feel unsafe when performing a job function, you can always refuse it.

When going through the stress of working under dangerous conditions, you should always take time to recharge. Take a step back from your assignment, take deep breaths, and allow yourself some time before going back to it. Taking some time off your assignment will give you time to rebalance your focus and concentration. You can also endeavour to stay out of conflicts with your colleagues and other people around you; the last thing you want to do is to get angry when you are already under a stressful situation, so stay away from conflict in every possible way.

Sometimes it looks impossible to avoid conflict at workplaces, but if it happens, try to manage it appropriately. It is not advisable for anyone to stay in a job that endangers their life or interferes with their peace of mind. If you cannot find another job immediately, try to comport yourself and manage the one you have now until you find a new one. Money is not always everything in life because when we get injured or sick from that job, depending on the level of damage, no amount of money can treat or save us.

Try not to always be perfect, as that will place you under pressure; anytime you do not fulfill that desire to perfect, you will began to stress out over it. Furthermore, always make yourself comfortable, and ease your tension in every possible way when carrying out your assignment. That way, you will not make costly mistakes that will jeopardize the job experience you have built over the years.

Chapter Sixteen
ANXIETY

ONE OF THE most common stressors people go through is anxiety over uncertainties regarding unknown things. People worry about the unknown; they live in fear of things they are not sure of. We often think: What if this happens? What if that happens? What will happen next? What will the reactions of people be? What will people say? Most of us worry about anything that crosses our minds; we worry about little things. Oftentimes, the things we worry about come out positively.

Many people worry about their job interviews, contract proposal presentations, what tomorrow will bring, and many other things. People have anxiety over what they cannot change and what they do not have control over in life. We should not worry about these things. When we worry in this way, we are drained and made less productive. If you observe closely, you will find out that anxiety affects us negatively because it makes us do things differently. And those things we do differently most times will not be beneficial to us—rather, they affect us in negative ways.

There is nothing positive about worrying over things we cannot control. All that is associated with anxiety is negativity, so it is imperative to reason wisely before getting worried over things unnecessarily, especially those things we cannot control. Anxiety has led many individuals to many health issues just because they could not control their emotions for the fear of the unknown. Many people have developed illnesses like heart attack, high blood pressure, and other dangerous medical conditions just because they get worried over things they could not control. This is not to say that worrying is inevitable—it's not. Yes, it's natural to get worried over things, but the extent or level we do it can be controlled by us.

Good coping strategy

Getting worried over things we are unsure of is natural, but we should always remember that eighty percent of what we worry about is imaginary. If we keep quiet about those things, they will most likely disappear. In life, we will be worried, we will be scared, we will get confused at some point along our journey. What we should understand is that getting worried about the things we are unsure of is not going to change anything. In fact, the more we get worried, the more we are exposing ourselves to bad health conditions that could be detrimental to us.

Worrying affects lots of things in our body—it reduces

the strength of our hormones, which will make us vulnerable to all kinds of illnesses. The less we worry about things, the better our physical body and mental health will function properly. One of the best and most effective ways to cope with anxiety is to take deep breaths. When we take deep breaths, our bodies get refreshed, and the anxiety we have within us tends to reduce.

Another thing that could help us with anxiety is getting enough sleep. Sleeping relaxes and strengthens our muscles, and when our muscles are relaxed, we are likely to perform well in our day-to-day living. When we are asleep, our anxiety, worries, fears, anger, and other things that disturb our bodies are temporarily silent, so getting enough sleep can reduce anxiety stress.

Meditation is another recommended way of coping with anxiety. When we give ourselves time to meditate, it relaxes us mentally. For meditation to positively impact our wellbeing, we should always meditate on the positive things of life. Let us not forget that positivity attracts positive things, while negativity also attracts negative things—so whichever we choose among the two is what will happen to us.

You should exercise regularly to release physical and mental weight. Exercising should not be a once-in-a-while thing—it's something you should be doing regularly and on an ongoing basis, to enable you get a positive result. When we exercise, we burn lots of calories, releases enzymes from our body, and pump more oxygen to our brain. When these three things happen to our body, our stress level decreases, and our life performances will begin to increase positively.

If exercising does not fully remove your anxiety, it will

certainly reduce it. Furthermore, spend time in a natural environment, such as the zoo, park, or beach, where you can see natural things like the sea, animals, and trees. Appreciating nature and looking at the great things God created on earth will make you feel good and will also give you hope for a better life. Having hope for a better life will wipe out your anxiety stress in no time. The pleasant surroundings and fresh air from the natural environment will help you relax and reduce your stress.

Additionally, engage yourself in helping other people. Feed the homeless or volunteer in your community to get yourself busy. When we are busy, we easily forget the things that are disturbing our minds. Finally, if you feel at any time your anxiety is getting out of control, you can seek out the help of a therapist who can walk you through more clinical ways of coping with anxiety.

Chapter Seventeen
RAPE

THERE ARE MILLIONS of rape cases reported yearly around the world, according to a recent statistic. Rape does not only happen to women—it happens to men as well. Raping a man or a woman is like taking their pride from them, and when people are raped, they will never be their normal self again, from the moment the act is committed against them. The aftermath of rape can be very damaging to the victims, so rape is not what anyone wants to experience. Rape can do so much damage to people. It can change their mindset, it can bring out the worst in them, it can have psychological effects on them, it can kill their trust of people.

Rape can make people contemplate or die by suicide. Many things can start to affect rape victims mentally; they may start to fear being alone; they may start to shut people out of their lives; they may start to fear crowded environments; and they may start to have fear of having sex with their partner or getting married. The mental and psychological effects and behaviour of rape victims can affect their children and people around them.

Rape stress on people cannot be over-emphasized because it can make a cool-headed person become violent. In the world today, many rape incidents are left unreported by some men and women for fear of been killed by the perpetrators. Some leave it unreported for fear of being ridiculed by their family and friends. When rape victims refuse to report their ordeals to the authorities, they are giving more power and strength to the people who perpetrated the act.

We should understand that rape does not just affect the victims alone—it affects their families, and all the people close to them. When we see or hear about anyone being a victim of rape, it is imperative that we report such cases to the authorities. Rapists should not be left loose on the streets; they should be placed where they rightfully belong, by law. If they are left to roam our streets without being penalized, they are likely to do more harm which will create more problems in society.

The more rapists we have on our streets, the more chaos and problem we will have in our society, so the earlier rape cases are reported the better for our communities. If you are a rape victim, do not be shy or scared to report the perpetrator. When you fail to report them, they are going to continue to do more harm to more people. In fact, you may be saving lives by reporting them to the authorities.

There are several rape cases where their victims are killed after the act. If you are lucky to be alive after a rape, it does not mean others will be lucky as you. Again, the stress of being raped can be devastating and can negatively change victims' lives forever. We should see reporting of attempted rape and rape cases as saving others' lives. If you refuse to make a report after being raped, you are likely to live with that burden, guilt, and agony for the rest of your life.

Good coping strategy

The stress of rape victims is very extreme and hard to cope with. The fact is when people are raped, certain things in them have been taken away—their pride is taken away, their trust is taken away, and their peace of mind is taken away. The first thing you want to do after the attack is to go to a safe place away from the attacker; the second thing is to speak to somebody you know that has a high level of integrity, preferably someone of the same gender. If you are a woman, talk to your mother, female friend, or female family members about your situation. And if you are a man, talk to your father or another man about it.

If someone of the same gender is not around you, look for anyone, regardless of gender, who has a high level of integrity, to talk to about your situation. Still, some people find it more convenient to open up to the same gender. It's understandable how hard the aftermath of rape can be, but we should try not to be scared. We should try to control ourselves; we should try to summon the courage to speak up because the more we try to suppress our feelings, the more negative impact the trauma can have on us.

Ask whoever you confided in to report your situation

to the authorities if you are too scared to do so yourself. But if they fail to do so, you should summon courage to directly report to the authorities on your own. Reporting to authorities can speed up your recovery process, knowing full well that the perpetrator has been brought to justice, and you will feel that you have saved others from being hurt by that same attacker.

Always have it at the back of your mind that when rapists get away with their crimes, they are likely to reoffend again by attacking other people. That is why it's important to use people in power to get them off the streets. Also, there are certain things you shouldn't do immediately after experiencing rape: You shouldn't change your clothes; you shouldn't shower right away; you shouldn't move or touch anything at the crime scene; and you shouldn't clean any parts of your body.

In the case of a rapist who has fled the crime scene, stay on the scene until first responders such as police and paramedics arrive. However, if the rapist is still on scene, move to a safe location before making any calls, for safety reasons. Sometimes rape cases are thrown out of court because of contaminated evidence. When investigators do not have a full analysis of evidence that can link rapists to the crime, the case can be thrown out of court, so it's very important to avoid doing any of those things mentioned above to avoid evidence contamination.

Do not allow shame, guilt, or threats from the perpetrator stop you from reporting your traumatic experience to the people close to you and the authorities. There are people you can seek support from, such as good family members and friends, people you know will not judge and condemn you because of your situation.

With time and therapy, the victim can certainly experience full recovery after such a traumatic encounter. With time and therapy, the things that happened to us will start to erase from our memories.

Chapter Eighteen
FACING DISCRIMINATION AND RACISM

DISCRIMINATION AND RACISM have contributed to the massive violence in the world today. In some countries, people are been discriminated against for who they are; some are by their sex, some are by their religion, some are by their disability, some are by their age, some are by their colour, some are by their race, and others are by their looks. Many individuals have been profiled against by the above examples. The stress that comes with discrimination and racism have affected millions of people around the globe.

Nobody deserves to be treated differently; every human being is created equally by God. When we face discrimination and racism, we tend to stress a lot over it. There are people who face these challenges on a daily basis so much so that they now think it's part of how they should live. No one should live under the stress of discrimination and racism because that stress could lead them to many health challenges, so they should not settle for it.

The effects of discrimination and racism get worse and more dangerous when you do not speak about it to anyone. Keeping your feelings to yourself will not only affect your self-esteem, it could also affect your social life. Discrimination is broader than racism because there is a lot associated with it; they face the same direction and describe elements of the same result, but there is still a thin line between discrimination and racism. This is not to make either of them more prominent than the other; they are both wrong.

Engaging in discrimination or racism can cause some people stray from their rightful path. So, before you discriminate or racially profile anyone, put yourself in their shoes. Would you be happy if someone else discriminated against or racially profiled you? If people can ask themselves this question before acting, most perpetrators will not even try to do it. Also, if they can empathize with the emotional and psychological effects of their actions on their targets, they surely will not proceed with it.

On the other hand, racism can be displayed in any form. It could be through jokes, it could be through costumes, it could be through slurs, it could be what is written on your shirt or dress, it could be through your body language or how you stare at someone. Some of the people that do these things to others might not completely know the tears or sorrow they are causing their victims. This is not to make excuses for them or to support their actions; often they do these things subconsciously. On the other hand, some of them know exactly the pain they are causing others.

Good coping strategy

Discriminating and being racist against other people is not new to us in our society. We all understand that discrimination and racism did not start today; it has been in existence even before many of us were born. The good news is that most nations in the world today frown at discrimination and racism. If you are going through discrimination or racism, save yourself the stress of underrating yourself before others or having low self-esteem just because of few people who fail to understand that everyone is created equal by God.

This is not to say that the negative effects of discrimination and racism are easy to control or live with, but there are ways we can manage it without any fighting or violence. Discrimination and racism are perpetrated by few people in our communities, and we should not use one bad egg among the good ones to judge everybody. What should give us strength and hope is the knowledge that such behaviours are not welcome in any society around the world.

Acts of discrimination and racism happen almost everywhere we go. They happen in our schools, restaurants, workplaces, and malls, just to mention a few. If you experience these acts in school, there are things you could do to manage the stress. Speak about your experience to people you know that does not possess that negative traits in them; do not just isolate yourself. Seek out people such as your professors, tutors, mentors, or your fellow students; this is a way of reducing your stress and isolation.

When you experience it in other public places, you could speak to your family members and friends about it. No matter where you experience discrimination or racism, just the follow similar approaches listed above and everything will be okay. The fact is that you are speaking up and not isolating yourself; when you isolate yourself, things get out of hand, but when you speak up there will be lasting solutions to the problem. Many people do not know that discriminating or being racist against others have serious penalties, and it is only when you speak up that they will face those penalties.

If you do not speak up, people around you will not know that such a thing is going on in your life. Speak up and involve people around you as well as those in power; this is when the appropriate solution can be provided for you. Further ways you can manage the stress is taking good care of yourself. Many people are quick to forget themselves because of the effects of discrimination and racism. We should not forget who we are and the way we used to take care of ourselves before our negative experiences. Taking care of yourself and looking good in front of the people looking down on you is one way of making the perpetrators stop their negative behaviour because when they realize what they are doing against you has no effect, they will back off.

This logic doesn't work in all cases, though. If this does not work in your own case, there are still several other approaches you could use to tackle the problem. Discrimination does not only happen between black, white, or brown people—it happens to all races in the world. It happens with black people, with white people, as well as brown people. For example, in some countries in Africa and Asia, some tribes do not intermarry with other tribes. What should we call this? Self-discrimination. This is another reason why we should not say we are the only victim when we experience it with other races because it happens in every race.

Another thing you could do is to educate yourself about these things; the examples above may have shown you some things you might not have known before now. When we educate ourselves about things that are bothering us, we may not react to them the way we do when we know nothing about these things. Not everybody who discriminates is racist against other people. There have been cases where white people advocate for black people, and there are cases also where black people advocate for white people.

Like we earlier discussed, discrimination and racism have been in existence even before we were born, and to curb discrimination and racism in our society, we need to work together as a team. Getting rid of discrimination and racism is possible, but it is not what one person, group, race or a particular country can eradicate alone. We need collective efforts from all sources and every human being to achieve that aim. Let it be known to everyone that there is no point fighting one another over one thing or the other because we all belong to one big family called the human race.

Chapter Nineteen
PANDEMIC

THE EFFECT OF a pandemic on the lives of individuals and communities can be immense any time it occurs around the world. The negative impact on lives can be disastrous. When a pandemic strikes in any country, it affects not only the people living in that country, but also the people living outside it as well. It also affects the country's economy. There are so many things a pandemic can affect, things like schools, businesses, finances, physical health, mental health, employment, relationships to mention a few. When these things are shut down or are affected, people will start to panic over the uncertainties of life and will begin to stress over it.

Pandemic season can be stressful and can create confusion among people. The fear of the unknown and what tomorrow may bring are what stresses people out more than the actual disease, especially when no vaccine has been found to treat it. The people that experience the stress of pandemic more are those whose family members are infected or taken away due to the virus. There are many cases where people are infected, and their family members deprived access to them. Imagine the stress they would go through after hearing their family member has been infected.

Imagine a father or mother going to work to try to put food on the table, only to have them find out they test positive for the virus. They will have to isolate, and neither their spouse nor children will be allowed to see them. Can you imagine the kind of extreme stress they will go through? Children not allowed to see their parents, husbands not allowed to see their wives, brothers or sisters not allowed to see their siblings. The scenarios above are extremely stressful to those going through them.

The stress that comes from pandemic restrictions affects family members who do not have the virus, just as much as it affects the infected persons. Not everyone can endure being prevented from seeing the people they love. Some family members may have stronger affection for some family members more than for other family members. The family members who feel stronger affection tend to go through more intense stress than those who feel less affection.

Good coping strategy

Going through times of uncertainty is hard, but it is not a life sentence, as many people may think. Only when we try to change the things we cannot change we go through extreme stress. We should understand that uncertainties are part of life and not something we can avoid; they are inevitable. A pandemic is a situation that does not only affect one person but everyone, so we are in the same boat together, and together we will all overcome it. There are many ways we can deal with the effects of deadly diseases, like the pandemic.

You should acknowledge that things can happen at any time and to always have an open mind for the uncertainties of life. There are some things you should limit doing all the time—things that trigger your mood when you do them too often. Limit the time you spend on social media as well as the time you spend watching the news. When you watch the news too often in pandemic season, it will certainly aggravate your stress level.

Watching too much news and spending too much time on social media reading about the infectious disease may allow more fear to grip us. This is not to say that watching the news and being on social media is entirely bad, but doing them too often in pandemic season is bad and will affect you. One thing we should not consider doing during pandemic season is giving up on life; we should always persevere and believe that things will get better.

Focus on the things you can control, and channel all your energy on things that are more productive instead of drowning yourself in thoughts of the unknown. We should always be optimistic no matter what we are going through in life. It is understandable that we all have limits to what we can take, but the hope of a better tomorrow should be what keeps us going. Take deep breaths, go hiking, meditate on positive things, read good books that focus on the positive things of life, and engage yourself in things that make you happy.

Before the COVID-19 pandemic, there have been other deadly diseases that have ravaged the world—for example, the Spanish Flu pandemic in 1918. When the Spanish Flu started, no one ever thought it would go away, but in time and with government guidance and directives about things we should and shouldn't do, the flu eventually subsided after two years.

When we follow the rules and regulations set out by our governments and adhere to all their restrictions, instructions, and recommendations—staying at home and isolating ourselves, quarantining after coming back from travel, using disinfectants, limiting our social gatherings, and maintaining good personal hygiene—things will eventually get back to normal.

This is not to say that the coronavirus will permanently go away; nor is it an assurance that it will disappear like the Spanish Flu. Rather it's an advisory that there is possibility that it will go away with the help of reliable vaccines in the future. Let us all have faith in God and keep our fingers crossed and hope for the best.

Chapter Twenty
LIFE AND CAREER STAGNATION

STAGNATION IS LACK of growth and development in the things we do. This can cause extreme stress for people who experience stagnation in their lives and careers. Stagnation is when we lose hope and interest in the things we used to love doing, when we don't move forward in life and remain in one position, when we suddenly stop setting goals for ourselves, when there is nothing exciting us anymore. People stress a lot when they experience stagnation.

When we stop pursuing our dreams, potentials, and other important things in life, that means we are experiencing stagnation. Sometimes, when people have tried everything within their power to move forward in life and nothing seems to be working out for them, they are experiencing stagnation. Being stagnant in life is so frustrating and stressful, especially when you have tried everything you could to step up your life and nothing is working.

There are different types of stagnation. One of them is when we have done everything to move forward and nothing is working for us. The other one is when we lose interest in doing things we love and that comes from within us. During a time of stagnation, we don't feel like doing things that will move us forward, and we lose total interest on them. Most times, it is after we have tried everything within our power to move forward and they did not work out. This is when we start losing feelings for or interest in these things.

There are other signs of stagnation in one's life and career. These signs mostly happen at work—for example, having no room for advancement or growth, having no increase in salary, being given tasks that surpass our abilities with no plans by the company we work for to train us on new things. These are just few examples of some of the things people experience at work that stresses them out.

Imagine working in a company where you have no hope of stepping up your position to earn more, or having qualifications and skills that your company's management does not recognize. Imagine applying for a position you know you are qualified for and that position is given to another employee who has less qualification and fewer skills. There is nothing more stressful when we experience any of the above examples. The above examples are signs of stagnation, bias, and favouritism in workplaces. When we start to see or experience things like these in our places of work, it is time to start thinking of looking for another job.

Good coping strategy

Stagnation is not a life sentence during which we have to continuously have regret and beat ourselves up. We are just required to make some changes to where we are and the things we do. When we make these changes, things will automatically change for us. Also, there is no point working in a place where there is no integrity or in a place where management is biased when making important decisions that could negatively impact the lives of their employees.

When we continue to work in places like these, our efforts and hard work will not be recognized, so it is time to move somewhere else. Jobs are not easy to come by, but being in a place where we are restless, stressful, and constantly unhappy is not worth it. There are some people in workplaces who don't get along with others; we have them as supervisors, we have them as managers as well as CEOs. When you come across these people, don't stress over their inability to get along with you because you cannot expect people who cannot even get along with themselves to get along with you.

Do not expect people to give you something they do not possess. Some people do not have love, care, and sympathetic feelings in them; they were not born with it. In addition, some people were born with it, but due to one trauma or the other they lost those feelings within them. So, do not expect people that lack self-love and feelings for others to give them to you.

We should understand that people cannot give us the things that are not built inside of them, things they do not have. Never try to change or control what people do, believe in, or say. When you try to do that, you are creating room for stress and making things difficult for yourself. Always remember that you are who you want to be, and all you need to do is to put in more effort and focus on that thing you are aspiring to become.

Some people find solace in helping other people. If you are one of those people, you could work towards a career that advocates for victims going through the same problems you had. When you do that, you will definitely feel less stress knowing full well that you will now be working closely with people going through similar stressors that you once went through.

Chapter Twenty-One
UNFORGIVENESS

HAVING AN UNFORGIVING heart towards other people is incredibly stressful. When we do not forgive and let go of things that hurt us, they will continue to hurt us. Before discussing how unforgiveness can hinder us from moving forward in life and how it could kill us slowly, let us discuss the story about the unforgiving snake and the machete:

There once was a snake crawling through the bush in a village. A sharp machete was on the ground, and when the snake crawled on the machete, the machete slightly hurt the snake. The snake was very furious at the machete. Out of anger and unforgiveness, the snake rolled itself around the machete and began to squeeze it. The snake did not realize that what it was squeezing was a sharp machete.

The snake squeezed and squeezed the machete out

of revenge and anger, believing that it was hurting the machete but not knowing that it was hurting itself. The more the snake squeezed the machete, the more the snake was hurting itself. After squeezing around the machete for an exceedingly long time, the snake got more severely hurt and died in the process.

That is the same way humans hurt themselves when they do not forgive the people who wronged them. When we do not forgive the people who have wronged us, we will continue to feel the hurt in our hearts. The more we harbour grudges in our hearts, the more they damage us. Forgiving those who have wronged us is like setting ourselves free from that bondage and stress.

You don't have to associate with people that hurt you after forgiving them; you can set your boundaries with them or give them distance as a precautionary measure to gird your heart from being hurt again. The most important thing is that you have forgiven them wholeheartedly. Many would ask: How do we know we have forgiven someone? The three ways we acknowledge that we have forgiven someone is that we are no longer bitter over what they did to us, not angry whenever we see them, and not using the thing they did to us against them in any way.

There are several signs when we don't fully forgive those who wronged us. Some of these signs are: not being happy when we see them; still feeling stressed and bitter in our hearts whenever we think about what they did to us; not protecting them from things that could hurt them when we see them in danger. These are the signs of unforgiveness that can hinder us from having peace of mind. Many people stress over not forgiving the people that wronged them in their day-to-day life.

When you hold on to the wrongs people did to you, it is like holding on to the past, and when you hold on to your past, you will remain in that past and you cannot move forward. But when you let go, you will gain that automatic freedom, and your life will begin to move forward. Holding on to those grudges will not only hinder you from progressing in life, it will also turn you into an angry and bitter person. When we are angry and bitter, we go through extreme stress that could jeopardize our lives.

If we fail to forgive those who wronged us, we are drowning ourselves in thoughts of anger, hate, resentment, and vengeance. When we have these negative thoughts in our heads, we will become unproductive and stressed, and we may develop anxiety and depression which could lead us to chronic health problems.

Good coping strategy

The first thing we should do when we have unforgiving spirits in us is to pray to God to develop that positive forgiving spirit in us, to forgive those who have wronged us. Only God can plant the spirit of forgiveness in you. Many people think that when they forgive other people that they are helping those people. The truth is when you forgive those that wronged you, you are actually helping yourself, not them.

Anyone who forgives other people's wrongdoings is setting themselves free from that bondage that could hinder them from moving forward in life. Several bible verses talk about forgiveness. Let's look at some of them:

God also stated in Luke 6:37: "Judge not, and you will not be judged; condemn not, and you will not be condemned; forgive, and you will be forgiven." This means that whatever we do to others, God will do to us.

When we forgive, we will reap the benefits of that forgiveness. There is a quote that says, "Forgiveness is a gift you give to yourself." What does this really mean? It simply means that when we set ourselves free from anger, bitterness, hatred, and unforgiveness, we are actually helping ourselves to move forward because when we hold on to these negative feelings of unforgiveness, we may remain stagnant for the rest of our lives.

Unforgiveness is like an object that is mounted on one spot and doesn't move. If you hold on to something that stays in one position, you will definitely remain in that spot with that thing, with no chance of moving forward. But if you let loose and let go, you will now be free from the chains and every hindrance holding you to that thing in that one spot.

Another bible verse we could look at is Luke 17:4: "And if he trespasses against you seven times in the day, and turns to you seven times, saying, 'I repent,' you must forgive him." This means that it does not matter the number of times people wrong us—there is no maximum number of times we can forgive. We must continue to forgive people that wrong us all of the time.

Additionally, in Colossians 3:13, we are told, "The Lord has forgiven you, so you also must forgive." The lesson here is that we forgive others because God forgave us. The bottom line is if God can do it, we also should be able to do it. There are so many other bible chapters and verses that teach us about forgiveness, and we can go on and on through them, but for now we will only use the above three verses as illustrations about the benefits of forgiveness.

When we forgive others, we are saving ourselves from extreme stress, potential depression, anger, anxiety, and hostility. If we refuse to forgive people who wrong us, we are exposing ourselves to severe depression, mental health issues, and even post-traumatic stress disorder (PTSD). Finally, forgiving people who have wronged us does not only put us right with God, it also reduces our stress and gives us the peace of mind we always crave.

Chapter Twenty-Two
POVERTY

IN THE WORLD today, poverty stress has affected so many families in different forms and ways. There are several types of poverty, but in this chapter, we will only look at three of them. The first one is generational poverty, the second one is situational poverty, and the third one is absolute poverty.

Generational poverty is when people come from a poor family background, meaning their family has been living in poverty before they were even born. Situational poverty, on the other hand, is when people were once financially comfortable, but circumstances or situations brought them down to live in poverty. Absolute poverty, also known as abject poverty, is when people literally live from hand to mouth, with no good food, no good clothes, no clean water, no good shelter, and no proper education.

Abject poverty is not common in Western countries; it is mostly common in Third World countries. People living in abject poverty go through extreme stress because most of them do not even know where their next meal is coming from. Abject poverty derives from generational poverty, which is inevitable, but situational poverty can be avoided and controlled; there can be hope of getting back on our feet after we overcome the circumstances that put us in situational poverty.

Many people who are in situational poverty today did not plan to be in this state, but circumstances beyond their control brought them into it. Living in abject poverty stresses many people around the world. Poverty stress is not what anyone wants to go through in life or would wish for someone else. There are so many negative conditions associated with abject poverty; some of these conditions include homelessness, lack of money, inadequate healthcare, lack of nutritious food, lack of good clothing, living in unsafe neighbourhoods and environments, etc. We can go on and on with the list of things poverty can cause.

Sometimes poverty can affect how long someone will live, depending on the severity of the impact of poverty on them. Poverty forces people to live in an uncomfortable position and a place that gives them restlessness. There is poverty in many nations, especially in Third World countries, as earlier mentioned above, where leaders care less about their citizens' welfare. Many have died, and some have critical health conditions due to lack of money to take care of themselves.

These people live in constant fear and worry of where their next meal will come from. People living in poverty go through constant stress every day, not knowing what tomorrow may bring for them. The stress associated with poverty has torn many families apart by creating family violence within them. Stress of poverty has made some peace-loving people become violent in their families. If people living with the stress of poverty do not get help on time with their financial struggles, they may end up having physical, mental, and psychological health problems or use the wrong coping strategies.

When we see people living in poverty, it is imperative to give them helping hands to ease their pain because showing kindness to strangers can ease their pains and change their lives. Many parents living with the stress of abject poverty always have unnecessary guilt in them for not being able to provide for their families. Some of them experience problems with memory, problems with concentration, and loss of interest in their favourite hobbies.

Additionally, they might even experience moodiness, withdrawal from the public, have high and low mood fluctuations, deal with sleeplessness, as well as suicidal thoughts or a desire to self-harm. The above examples are the things poverty stress could do to people. Poverty stress can prevent us from using our social opportunities, affect our family relationships, and can also stop us from attaining our full potential.

As poverty affects parents, so it affects their children. The effects on children are more intense but is based on their level of maturity. Poverty stress affects children's wellbeing, academic performance, and social life—and it could even steal their childhood from them. Children do not fully understand how poverty affects them until they are of a certain age. And when they come to the realization of how poverty is affecting them, some of them may understand the situation but some might not—especially those that have friends who come from rich families. Those that do not understand their parent's plight of poverty might became rude and disrespectful to them, while those who do understand the condition of their parents may be supportive to them.

It all goes back to how the children were nurtured and brought up, as well the people they associate with, their level of understanding, and how they perceive the things of life. The stress poverty places on parents' shoulders cannot be compared with that of their children's; regardless of how difficult things may be for parents, they will still have to go out there through thick and thin to provide for their children. Good parents living in abject poverty deserve accolades for not giving up on themselves as well as their dependents because not all parents have the strength to persevere through such difficult times.

Good coping strategy

Living in poverty is one of the most difficult situations in life, but it is not a life sentence or the end of the world. Poverty might seem endless to many families, but if proper planning is implemented, it could eradicate poverty permanently from their lives. It might not be your fault that you were born into abject poverty, but if you remain in that abject poverty, it becomes your fault. There are several things you could do to cope with poverty and change your situation. Most people living in abject poverty are still in it because of lack of proper planning and education.

This is not to put blame on them that they refused to go to school; the fact is many of them didn't have the finances to take up that task of studying in school because their main focus was on what they would eat to stay alive. Getting proper education can turn things around for people living in abject poverty.

The other thing you could do is try digging deep into your family background on how they handled money. Did they have good spending habits, or were they extravagant in their day-to-day life? There are cases of people who were once rich and later became broke due to money mismanagement. Read books about money, and do your research about profitable investments to learn more about how you can invest in them. Once you have that knowledge, utilize what you have learned to change your mind set about money. Stop the habit of buying things you don't need; when you do that you are wasting the money you could have wisely invested in a profitable business that can fetch you more money.

In some cases, people buy things they do not need to impress people that do not even like them. Try to do things at the right time, and stop copying the lifestyles of others by trying to do whatever they are doing when you are not ready for it. Live below your earnings, and never increase your financial obligations when you are not fully ready to do so. Examine your circle of friends and investigate things that trigger you to spend your money unnecessarily.

If you find yourself doing things because your friends are doing it, break out from that circle and make new friends that do not spend money extravagantly. That way you will be able to save more money, which you can invest on investments that are profitable. In no time, poverty will be a thing of the past in your life and that of your family. If at some point you feel more worried about things not working out or towards your expected direction, do not struggle alone in silence. Take advantage of other resources that talk about good spending habits, profitable investments, and lucrative businesses available to you where you can learn more techniques to financial freedom.

Chapter Twenty-Three

LOW SELF-ESTEEM

AT ONE POINT or another in our lives, some of us have experienced the stress of low self-esteem. When we don't feel good about ourselves in the things we do, this is a sign of low self-esteem. When we see ourselves as incompetent, unworthy, unlovable, and unacceptable in society, these too are signs of low self-esteem.

Most people who have low self-esteem have experienced physical, emotional, or psychological abuse. Other people who experience low self-esteem are those who are overweight and those that are physically challenged.

In addition, other signs of low self-esteem include difficulty speaking up, difficulty making our own choices, and difficulty prioritizing our own needs and feelings over the needs and feelings of other people. People go through the stress of low self-esteem because they do not have the courage to do things others are doing, and instead of forcing themselves to do the needful, they resign to stressing over them. Low self-esteem can limit people from setting boundaries between themselves and those hurting them on daily basics.

Low self-esteem could make the most active people to become inactive in their day-to-day life. People with low self-esteem find it difficult to interact with other people, and they also find it difficult to work together in groups. That feeling of looking down on themselves constantly stresses them out, and they find it difficult to appreciate themselves even if they have done well more than others. Some people who are a little overweight find it difficult to feel good in whatever they wear. Each time they want to go out, they change their clothes many times until they feel comfortable with what they are wearing.

Low self-esteem stress is awfully bad for people to have because it can negatively impact their growth in society, and it can limit them from reaching their full potential in life. People with low self-esteem stress are mostly behind in whatever they do because they always have that spirit of withdrawing from the public. Most of them do not want to be seen at the forefront of any activity; they prefer peeping from behind their peers.

When they are in school, they don't want to answer any questions first, even when they know the answer, and when they are involved in outside school activities, they don't want to be the first to try things out. They always have the habit of doing things after everyone else has done them. If low self-esteem is not taken care of, it can lead people to depression, bad coping strategies, and other health issues. Most of them prioritize other people's needs over their own. They spend their hard-earned money buying things for people in order to please them and to be able to feel good about themselves.

Making other people feel good is what boosts them to feel good about themselves. This is not to say that buying things for people or helping them is bad, but when you do it due to your low self-esteem, it becomes a problem. When people who have low self-esteem don't change their circle of friends who bring out the worst in them, over time their condition might change from bad to extremely critical one. Always remember that "a stitch in time saves nine," meaning that if we correct our mistakes on time or fix things that are affecting us early on, it could save a whole lot of trouble for us later.

Good coping strategy

The majority of people have experienced low self-esteem stress in one way or the other. These experiences of low self-esteem are mild for some people and intense for others. We should take total control of our lives by trying to understand what low self-esteem is, its causes, by educating ourselves about it. When we know the causes of our problems and how they affect us, there is possibility of finding lasting solutions to it. Having that knowledge can give us the strength to generate ideas on how to solve those problems. Making that change of overcoming the stress of low self-esteem starts with you.

Only you understand yourself better than any other person does, so for that change to be possible, you must initiate it. Stay connected with people who encourage you and make you feel important, and isolate yourself from those who bring out the worst in you. The circle you are in can determine how well you will perform in society. If you stay under the influence of bullies and those who talk down on you or other people around you, you may not recover from that low self-esteem—and it is also likely that you will become a bully too.

Try to do things with your conscious mind, and ignore triggers from your subconscious mind. Live in the moment, and do not worry about other things around you or about your future. For people who are overweight, and those with disabilities, always remember that you are not the one who created yourself. Don't forget that there are lots of people out there that are in worse situations than you. So, do not always assume you have the worst problems in the whole world. Even if your case is the worst, there is still a solution to it because there is absolutely no problem without a solution.

Please note that problems would not exist if there were no solution to them. Solutions are always there, but we are too blind to see them most times. That is why it is imperative to think positively in whatever we do because positive thinking attracts positive things, while negative thinking attracts negative things. What we give out of ourselves is exactly what we get back, so if we think that something is not good, we should not expect that good things will come out from it. It is only when we have that positive spirit that things will happen to us positively.

Let us always exhibit that positive attitude so that whatever we do or whatever we are going through will come out positive for us too. Low self-esteem should not take the better part of you. You shouldn't be so engrossed with negative feelings and deprive yourself of the good feelings of life. You are not alone in this. Anytime you feel that things are beyond your control or the good coping strategies outlined above are not working, there are other resources out there you could use. Seek out a therapist or psychologist who specializes in resolving extreme low self-esteem problems to enable you conquer that stress permanently.

Chapter Twenty-Four
DOMESTIC VIOLENCE

DOMESTIC VIOLENCE HAPPENS every second in many families around the world today, and a high percentage of people in different communities have all experienced domestic violence in one form or the other. Women are most vulnerable to domestic violence, more than men; they are often and easily overpowered and battered by men. This not to say that men are not vulnerable or go through domestic violence as well, but women have higher percentage of it. Regardless, the fact is domestic violence is not what anyone should go through.

Many lives have been lost due to domestic violence. Any form of violence should not be tolerated from anyone, be it a man or woman. There are two major types of domestic violence: physical violence and psychological violence. This violence normally occurs when one person tries to take total control of the other person. And when that person refuses to comply with the wish of the other person, that is when they become violent to that other person who resists them.

Domestic violence does not just affect those who are directly involved in it—it affects their entire family. There are lots of reasons we should not accept any form of violence in our homes. When we are violent in front of our children or any young child, there is possibility that when they grow up, they too will be violent to their partners when they get married or violent to their peers outside their home. There is an idiom that says, "monkey see, monkey do." This is not just a mere saying—it is a truth that some people refuse to understand and believe.

Anything you do in front of your children, they will copy that same behaviour and apply it to anyone they come across. That is why many children exhibit similar characteristics of their parents when they grow up. Whatever you nurture them with at a young age, they will give back to you and society. The stress of domestic violence is not easy to cope with because it drains us by taking the better part of us. When we are passing through domestic violence, we lose our senses, concentration, and the ability to function properly in society.

When your partner aggressively insults you or threatens you after resisting their attempts to control you, this is domestic violence. Their acts of violence against you could lead you to having extreme stress, low self-esteem, anxiety, depression, and post-traumatic stress disorder if you don't put an end to it or seek the help you need. When that happens, it could affect your whole life and that of your children. Oftentimes, domestic violence leaves physical scars, broken hearts, and psychological and emotional effects.

Sometimes it takes an exceedingly long time for victims of domestic violence to recognize and report it. Perpetrators of domestic violence most times isolate their victims from where they believe they could possibly get help, such as their family members, friends, social places, and any resources. And when their movements are restricted, their stress level becomes more intense. In addition, there are various health problems that may arise from the stress associated with domestic violence; be mindful of them.

Good coping strategy

Coping with domestic violence is incredibly challenging and difficult, especially when we love the perpetrator more than they love us. One thing you should understand is that in domestic violence, we should put love aside and face reality. When somebody is violent against us, most of the time they have lost their feelings for us because if they genuinely loved us, they wouldn't physically or emotionally hurt us intentionally.

You should always put sentiments aside when it comes to your safety and the safety of the people you love. Remember, you do not have to fight this alone. There are so many resources you can use to cope with the stress or eradicate those awful feelings. The worst thing you can do to yourself is to try to conceal what you are going through. If your partner tries to restrict you from seeing the people you love, try to break out from that chain of bondage to see those people that can help you out of that situation.

Sometimes, common hugs and words of encouragement can go a long way in reducing your stress. You must break yourself loose and take the first step by allowing someone to guide you through the right path to lasting solutions to your problems. Never accept domestic violence or get comfortable with it as a way of life. Speak up and get people involved so that appropriate solutions can be found for you. Do not allow anyone to try to force you to accept any act of violent behaviour against you as normal. Involve appropriate authorities on time to save you from your predicament, pain, and agony. Always remember that most victims of domestic violence who delayed reporting their ordeals to the authorities never live to tell their story.

There are some domestic violence situations where victims are restricted or isolated from their family, friends and the public by the person who is violent against them. They strip them off all means of communications to prevent them from getting the help they need. If you fall into that category, your life is terribly in danger and there are couple of things you could do to break free. One of them is to remain calm with the violent person, and the second one is to comply with whatever they tell you to do. That way you will make them feel comfortable and build some trust. When they believe and feel in control of you, they will likely loosen some of the restrictions placed on you.

Some of these loosened restrictions could be access to a phone or computer or perhaps allow you to go for a walk or to a grocery store with them. When you have access to the above examples, play smart and quickly send private message to the people you know can help you, people who know your complete address and phone number. The message don't have to be too long, a simple message like " I'm in danger at home, please call the police" if the perpetrator has any weapon in their possession, also state it, " he has a knife or gun" or any weapon you know he has.

This is important because the police need to know, so that they can better prepare for the assignment ahead of them. If you have the opportunity to go outside with him, comport and relax yourself until you find someone you believe can physically restrain them to enable you escape to a safer location where you can call for help. If they have any weapon there on them, you also have to inform the person who is trying to help you, when you don't let them know, you are endangering their life too. On the other hand, when the person who is been violent against you did not restrict you from communicating or going out and you still feel that things are beyond your control and unsafe, you can seek help from one of the domestic violence agencies in your city or better still involve the authorities.

Chapter Twenty-Five

DISABILITY

LIVING WITH DISABILITY is one of the most stress-ful situations in life. There are several types and forms of disability. Disability could be physical, intellectual, or mental; it can affect vision, hearing, and more. The more difficult and intense your disability, the more it aggravates your stress level. Many people with disabilities find their situation unbearable. Some of them have died by suicide or attempted it, while others have simply resigned themselves to using bad coping strategies.

Physical disabilities are the disabilities people can see in you; other disabilities are invisible. It does not matter the kind of disability—the bottom line is that they affect many of us on a daily basis. When we are disabled, we tend to stress a lot about it, especially when we are dealing with the physical type of disabilities. The stress of disability can have huge negative impact on our personality and our day-to-day living. Disability can cause irritability, anxiety, low self-esteem, mood swings, and several other physical and mental health problems. Dealing with disability is one of the most difficult situations we could ever have.

When we have disability, some people in our society use it against us; they discriminate against us and make life unbearable for us. Life for people with disabilities will be much easier if able-bodied individuals assist them in one way or the other. Most times in our society some people do not seem to care much about people living with disability, except those who have a good heart and the fear of God. However, in many Western countries, the government always takes up the responsibility of taking care of people with disabilities; that care cannot be compared to Third World countries where most leaders are careless about their able-bodied citizens, let alone those with disabilities.

When we have disability, we feel different from other people and sometimes even feel like less of a human. Those negative feelings of stress inside of us make us feel insecure in our everyday lives and stresses us out on a daily basis. When we are living with disability, we may subconsciously start to act strange and weird towards ourselves and others or having the feelings of low self-esteem in the presence of others, which will allow our disability to overpower us. Regardless of how we got our disability or the nature of our disability, we shouldn't allow it to way us down in any way or affect the way we associate with others in our society. In addition, everyone deserves to feel good and comfort-able about themselves wherever they go or whatever they choose to do, without fear. We should freely, confidently, and comfortably study, work and do what we need to do in the society regardless of our disability status. And be able to stand against those who tries to make us uncomfortable or less of a human in the society. Anyone who tries to exhibit such negative character towards us or bully us because of our disability should be severely dealt with by the law.

Good coping strategy

Living with disability is not a death sentence or something you should constantly stress and worry about. The first thing you want to do when you have a disability is to accept your condition the way it is and take charge of your life. Do not try to be a denial because if you do that it is going to aggravate your stress level. Take absolute control of your life by doing things that make you happy; do not allow anyone to dictate to you how you should run your life because you know yourself better than them. You are the one wearing your shoes, and you know exactly where it hurts. No one knows you better than yourself; you know all the things that give you joy and make you happy, as well as those things that make you sad.

The second thing you want to do is to know your rights. When you know your rights, you can protect yourself by involving appropriate agencies anytime people discriminate against you. Not being knowledgeable about your rights can hinder you from taking appropriate action against those people who are trying to make you miserable. The good news is that many agencies frown at those trying to bully or take advantage of people living with disabilities by decisively penalizing them for their wrongful acts.

Many nations have created jobs that can accommodate people with disabilities and several other opportunities for everyone, regardless of their disability. Many countries have also enacted laws including equity acts to protect people living with disability. These measures taken by governments of many nations indicate people with disabilities are not alone in their situations. When you take into account the above explanation of how people with disabilities have been protected, you will understand that you are never alone in your situation.

Most times knowing that we are not alone in our situation gives us the courage and strength to move on in life. Your disability should not be a barrier to your life or stop you from reaching your potential. Always remember that our situations can mold us and shape us, but they should not define us or determine who we will become. It is okay to feel different among our peers or other people. It is okay to have difficulty with things we do due to our disabilities, but that should not stop us from doing the things we love. Your happiness is in your hands; you should not expect or depend on other people to make you happy. However, if you are already depending on other people to be happy, you can make a change and that change starts with you.

People can make you laugh; people can get you excited; people can make you smile, but they cannot make you happy because happiness comes from within. Only you can ignite that light of happiness inside of you. Each time you are happy, your body brings out positive feelings that can make your day pleasurable. Never isolate yourself from the public; instead, surround yourself with people who inspire you, and do away with those who bring out the worst in you. Get rid of the self-pity that comes when you are not able to do things you could do before. Accept your life the way it is now.

Always remember that the only constant thing in life is change and that change can happen to anyone—anytime and anywhere. And when change happens in our lives, we should always summon the courage and strength to accept it because that ability to accept those changes is what will keep us moving forward. We may have been born with disability, or perhaps we got it in one way or the other after coming to this world. But that should not hinder us from our dreams and aspirations.

Resources have been created in several ways by the government for people living with disabilities, where they can explore ways to reach their full potential in life. To be sad sometimes is not something you can always resist or avoid; even able-bodied people feel sad too, sometimes. However, you can set a time limit to feel these emotions on your own, but it shouldn't be on daily basis. Your goal should be to always have reasons to be happy. Each time you do not feel happy, think about those positive things in your life that will ignite those feelings of happiness within you.

Sometimes, it is okay to be sad because suppressing feelings of sadness may hinder you from healing emotionally. So, experiencing those feelings of sadness sometimes may give you the strength you need and will reenergize you to further deal with or manage your situation. This is not to say that being sad is a good thing to do, but if it is something that will positively

strengthen us to manage our situation, then it becomes a Good coping strategy. Look for exercises that are within your restrictions; find ways to do these exercises because they will help you in both your physical and mental health.

Do not feel that the world has come to an end just because you have a disability. There are several other things that you are blessed with that you should be grateful for, things that others do not have. If for any reason you find it difficult to manage your disability with your current job, retrain for a profession that will accommodate your disability more; that way your stress will reduce, and you won't have to worry much about life.

Chapter Twenty-Six
UNHAPPINESS

WHEN WE DO things that we are not pleased or satisfied with, it is a sign of unhappiness. There are several things that can make us unhappy in life; most of these things are the things we do on daily basis. Sometimes, being unhappy does not have anything to do with the things we do, but the unhappiness has to do with our impulses as well as our inner feelings. Each time we are unhappy, we tend to stress over it a lot, and this can negatively impact how well we perform in our daily lives.

Some of the things that can cause unhappiness is not getting enough sleep. Sleep is very essential to your health, and when you don't get enough of it, it affects your entire body system which could result in unhappiness. Another thing that could negatively impact your happiness is when you live in your past. Living in your past experiences always affects your present and conscious mind. When we bring our bad past experiences into our conscious minds, they tend to make us unhappy and stressed.

Feeling lonely is another thing that could stress you out. This feeling of loneliness does not mean you do not have anyone in your life. In most cases those people in your life are not filling that empty vacuum you have and are making you more miserable. Sometimes, you may have friends, partners, and family members all around you and still feel unhappy and lonely. This happens when all these people around you are not playing their rightful roles in your life. They always bring out the worst in you and never see anything good or positive in you.

These kinds of people are toxic in your life and will never make you move forward. When you don't move forward, that is when you become unhappy and stressed. That is why it is imperative to know as much information as possible about the people around you before drawing them close. The only two sure ways to know them is through our inner feelings and with time, but most times we don't listen to our inner feelings because we get carried away with the blood ties of family, long-time friendships, or people's physical looks.

When we are blinded or carried away by the above examples, it will be more difficult to know their true colours or identities. This is not to say that all family members, friends, and neighbours are all bad people because there are some around us who are truly good and make us feel happy. But sometimes they also tend to be the cause of our problems. When you are lucky to have good people around you, never let them go because they are not easy to find. Furthermore, some people think that having all the good things in life will make them happy, but what they do not realize is that material or worldly things can only give them temporary excitement, not permanent happiness.

There are millions of people out there who have all the good things in life, and they still lack happiness. Happiness is not what we can buy with money: it is something that comes from inside of us, and sometimes happiness comes from the good we do to others. Other things that could attract unhappiness is blaming yourself about things that are beyond your control and comparing yourself to others. There are some things in life we do not have control over, and when these things happen to us, we tend to try to change them, forgetting that they are beyond our control. It's when we try changing things beyond our control that we become unhappy.

Another pitfall is comparing yourself to other people. Remember that we all are created differently, and the things you can do are not what the other person can do. If you understand that everyone has things they are good at and things they are not good at, this will save you from the stress of unhappiness.

Good coping strategy

The first thing to do on the journey to happiness is knowing God first—and not just knowing him, but also believing in him wholeheartedly. Only God can give you that inner peace you always crave. Most times it is what we feel inside of us that makes us happy, and that positive feeling inside of us is the spirit of God. In addition to knowing God truthfully, another thing that can make us happy is what we put out to the world. Happiness is not always what we do for ourselves or what we get from others; sometimes it is what we do for other people who are in need that gives us happiness as earlier mentioned above.

Smiles are contagious; when we smile, we can put a smile on someone else's face—and we get the positive reflection of our own smile right away. When we make people happy, we get similar feelings right back. Making other people happy is like making ourselves happy as well. For example, when you give somebody free gifts, you will see the smile on their face, and since that smile is infectious you are likely to smile back at them. If you have everything in life and you are still not happy, it's time to seek the face of God and start doing good things for people. Without God's presence in your life, you will always lack that inner peace.

Always put God first in whatever you do, and every other thing will follow, as the bible says in Matthew 6:33: "Seek ye first the kingdom of God, and his righteousness, and all these things shall be added unto you." This means that when we put God first in our lives, every other good thing in life will be added unto us, including the happiness we always crave. Other things you can do while placing God first in your life is volunteering in community services to help in ways that will be beneficial to other people rather than to ourselves.

You could also go out on your own to feed the poor, clothe them, and render help to the people you feel need it. Do not wait for them to ask before doing it; do it anytime your spirit leads you to. If you feel led in your spirit that they need that help, render it to them right away.

Learn to take deep breaths each time you are stressed out, and exercise regularly because exercises lowers stress hormones and also improves sleep quality.

Spend time in nature, and always think about positive things to be grateful for in your life. The way bad things are happening to us is the same way good things are happening to us too. We should always think about the good things that have happened to us and be grateful for them and not always think about the bad experiences that keep drowning us in pain and agony.

Remember, always put God first in whatever you do, and every other good thing will follow according to the declaration of the bible in Matthew 6:33, as mentioned above.

Chapter Twenty-Seven
GUILT

THE FEELING OF guilt is not what anyone wants to experience. However, in one way or the other we have all experience the feeling of guilt in our lives. Experiencing guilt does not necessarily make us a bad person; most times it is something we did subconsciously that keeps haunting us day by day. It could be simple things, like not giving the perfect directions to strangers who missed their way, grabbing the last piece of pizza, making uncomplimentary remarks about someone else, losing your patience, not allowing an elderly person in front of us at check-out counters, or not rendering helping hands to somebody who fell down, and so many other scenarios that could make us feel guilty.

We always have the stress of guilt when we do these

things or fail to do them at the appropriate time. Guilt is a terrible burden that can continue to reflect in our minds and memories if not taken care of. We feel the stress of guilt when we think we did not do the right thing. Feelings of guilt can make the body not function properly, which could result in headaches, over-thinking, bitterness, anger, and nightmares. The stress of guilt can drain you and take the best part of you if it gets out of control.

Other things that could attract feelings of guilt are things like refusing to speak the truth when you know it, taking something that does not belong to you, lying to your parents or someone who has been truthful to you all their life, cheating in an exam hall, faking things when you know they are not true, and so on. It is virtually doing any wrong things to people that brings us feelings of guilt.

Not everyone has remorse or feelings of guilt after doing wrong things to others. There are some people who will wrong you and will not feel that guilt in them. Do not be perplexed when you come across such people; always remember that it is what people have in them that they can give to others. Some people do not have those feelings of guilt at all in them; that is why when they wrong anyone, they do not feel that they have done anything wrong. This is not to make excuses for their bad behaviours—it is just a heads-up for you to know that there are people who will not have remorse or feelings of guilt after their wrongdoing to you and others. It's what is inside of us that we can also give to others, so if we don't have that spirit of guilt in us after doing something wrong, there is no way we will show that remorse or feel guilty when we are wrong.

The stress of guilt only happens to those who have that

remorseful spirit in them. Being remorseful after offending people or doing something wrong will not only restore your peace of mind, it will also afford you the opportunity to amend your bad ways and wrongful acts against others.

Good coping strategy

The first thing you should do when you realize you have done something wrong is to acknowledge that mistake, as well as understand that no one is perfect in life. Feelings of guilt remind us that we have an ethical and good moral standard of life. When we feel guilty, our spirit is telling us to make amends and change our ways. It is good for normal human beings who have done something wrong to others to have a remorseful spirit of guilt in them. It is okay to feel bad when you realize that you have wronged other people, and that feeling of guilt is a sign that you have remorse over what you did wrong. When you find out that you have done something wrong, always find a way to put the situation right, but if it's too late to correct that mistake, learn from it so that you won't make a similar mistake next time.

If you did something that affects someone else, apologize to them and make them understand that it was not an intentional act. Apologizing to them shows that you have empathy and will also make that person you have wronged realize that there are still good people around who can admit their mistakes no matter the consequences. Admitting your mistakes will give you the opportunity to learn from them, which will make you do better next time. Not admitting those mistakes and suppressing them inside of you is what will get you into more trouble because you will feel that it is okay to hide your mistakes.

It is not good to repeatedly continue to do wrong things to people when we know they are wrong. Try making up for every wrongdoing to others, no matter how hard it may seem for you. Age does not count—even if the person you have wronged is a young child, you still owe them that apology. Every one of us knows right from wrong, so each time we do something wrong we will definitely know it. There is no point shying away or blaming your wrongful acts on your mood, impulses, or other people. You should always take responsibility for your wrongdoings.

Taking responsibility for the things you have done wrong may make you look bad on the outside and in the sight of other people, but on the inside it is actually shaping you to be a better person in life. In some cases, the stress of guilt is more intense when the person you offended is not physically present for you to apologize to, especially if you really prefer to do that apology in person. For example, perhaps the injured party angrily left the scene and did not give you a chance to apologize. Or perhaps your offence occurred long ago, and the person you offended died before you could apologize. When you find yourself in one of these situations, know that you don't have to live in the agony of guilt for the rest of your life—all you need to do is to confess your sins wholeheartedly to God through his son Jesus Christ and repent of them completely.

God's word in the bible says, "If we confess our sins, he is faithful and just to forgive us our sins, and to cleanse us from all unrighteousness." (1 John 1:9) God is the only one that can forgive us our sins and restore our peace of mind in the absence of those we have offended.

Chapter Twenty-Eight
OVERWEIGHT/OBESITY

THE CAUSE OF obesity, generally, is the consumption of too many foods and not having any plans of burning the calories consumed. We may begin to experience obesity when we do the following: lying down immediately after eating, heavy consumption of sugary food, high consumption of fatty foods, eating late at night, and eating too frequently. The stress of obesity has affected many individuals around the world. When we are overweight, we tend to restrict ourselves from so many activities.

We withdraw ourselves from socializing with friends and other people in society, and sometimes we even isolate ourselves from family members and stop doing the things we once loved. We always create that belief within ourselves that we are not good enough to be seen outside or that people will laugh at us. Then we will begin to have sleepless nights and nightmares, and start to develop that self-hate in our minds. When we develop the habit of condemning ourselves before others, then we will start to have low self-esteem, which will further complicate our situation and make us stress more.

Obesity could be hereditary too, meaning that you could get it from either of your parents or your lineage. If you got your obesity from your family, that means it is beyond your control. Oftentimes, when things are beyond our control, we stress about them a lot, forgetting that it's not within our power to change the situation. In the case of hereditary obesity, we don't have that ability to change our situation, and all we really need to do is to learn how to live and manage our condition.

The stress of obesity could lead you to many health problems like stroke, diabetes, heart diseases, breathing problems, sleep apnea, and many other health challenges. There are some illnesses that could lead you to obesity, as well as some drugs that could make you become obese. That is why it's imperative to be careful not to use bad coping strategies that will involve the use of dangerous drugs that could lead you to obesity during your stressful times. Additionally, there are no clothes that you will feel comfortable wearing when you are overweight because you may either assume they are too small or too big because of your low self-esteem. That stress of overweight and the assumption that your clothes are not fitting properly may continue to haunt you each time you are about to go out, unless you take decisive measures to end those negative thoughts.

Good coping strategy

Coping with the stress of obesity is not an easy task; it requires determination and consistent efforts. The first thing you should do when coping with the stress of obesity is to accept yourself the way you are. There are some things we should not consider doing when we are living with obesity, and we shouldn't condemn or look down on ourselves before anyone. Sometimes, how we present ourselves will influence the way other people will treat us. Your condition may shape and mold you, but you should not allow it to define who you are or affect the way you do things.

When you allow your condition to take total control of you, it will take the better part of you. Avoid the habit of self-isolation from friends, family, and the public, and incorporate good stress-relief strategies into your daily life. Being overweight is not a life sentence that you should continue flogging yourself over emotionally. There are lots of stress-relief programs you can engage yourself in to manage your situation, so all hope is not lost. Engage yourself in regular physical activities and develop healthy eating habits with food that will not place you at risk of other health challenges.

Surround yourself with good and supportive friends, family members and positive people who will encourage you in ways you can manage your condition. Practice the effective relaxation skills of deep breathing, stretching, yoga and other effective stress management activities available to you. Additionally, there are several other things you could do to manage your situation—things like distracting yourself from eating when you are not hungry, avoiding food you always crave, avoiding fatty and greasy foods, as well as eating foods that are low in fat.

If after trying the above coping strategies they don't seem to be working for you, you can seek the professional help of a counsellor who can walk you through how to be confident about yourself as well as other good coping strategies you could use to manage your stress and condition.

Chapter Twenty-Nine
SUICIDAL THOUGHTS

SUICIDAL THOUGHTS OR behaviours arise when we begin to nurture the ideas of taking our own life. When we are overwhelmed with these negative thoughts in our minds, it hinders our sense of reasoning, and all we can think of is to end everything by taking our lives. Suicidal thoughts come with lots of negative thinking and stress. We may start to think that life is worthless and hopeless. The stress of suicidal thoughts may push you to engage in activities that may be detrimental to your health. For example, you may start to abuse dangerous substances like hard drugs. You may also start to have feelings of guilt and loneliness.

Other things you may start doing include: isolating yourself from family and friends; exposing yourself to activities that will negatively impact your life; depriving yourself of sleep; feeling threatened by the presence of people. There are so many occurrences that can ignite suicidal thoughts in any individual, and these occurrences may vary. Suicidal thoughts can take over our minds after we have experienced extreme heartbreak, betrayal of trust, loss of someone very dear to us, and many other scenarios that could trigger our moods.

Many people drown themselves on a daily basis with thoughts of suicide when undergoing intense stress and depression. As you know, everyone is created differently— that is why we respond to stress in different ways. What stresses you out may not necessarily stress other people out. We all have different levels of resiliency in us, as well as varying abilities when it comes to resisting stress. In some cases, people will consider taking their own life only after they have exhausted every solution to their problem; others may consider suicide after minor difficulties in their lives.

Some people may have the solution to their problem right in front of them, but they are just too blinded by their emotional attachment to that problem, believing there is no way out. There are also some situations where people may have suicidal thoughts and not actually attempt carrying out suicide; others, regardless of the intensity of their stress level, will still attempt suicide. It all still channels back to individual's strengths and weaknesses when it comes to suicidal ideation.

The stress associated with thoughts of suicide causes us to fixate on our pain and will not allow us to see the positive side of things. We should always remember and have it at the back of our minds that there is no problem on earth without a solution, all we need to do is to not allow that problem take total control of our entire life.

Good coping strategy

The first step when coping with suicidal thoughts is the realization that our problem is not the worst thing that could happen to us, as well as understanding that there is no problem without a solution. If there is no solution to problems, those problems would not have existed in the first place—so, no matter how difficult and complicated our problems may be, there are always solutions to them. When you are on the brink of falling into thoughts of suicide, try the following to manage your situation:

Talk about your situation to someone who can help you. Reach out to good friends, family members, and those who can enlighten you about the importance of life, as well as how you can manage your stressful situation.

Look for things that will distract you from those negative thoughts. Develop a strategy of ignoring those thoughts whenever they strike your mind. One of the distracting techniques you could use is doing things you enjoy instead.

If you find it difficult to utilize the above coping strategies, take a long nap; when you wake up, more reliable coping techniques will come to your mind. Relaxing your brain will give you the strength and capability to function properly, and will allow you to make more reliable decisions to better your situation. Develop the habit of calling someone to come see you each time you are having difficulties dealing with the stress of suicidal thoughts. Listen to cool music that will positively boost your spirit, and read books about love, happiness, and joy.

Listening to cool music and reading books about positive things will trigger positive feelings which will circulate throughout your entire system to bring out the best in you. You could use other resources available to you, like the services of a therapist or psychologist, anytime you feel the above coping strategies are not working for you.

Chapter Thirty
REJECTION

WE ALL KNOW how we feel when we've been rejected for something we know deep down in our hearts we are qualified for, or something we know we are entitled to, or something we believe we are entitled to. There are some people who have experienced rejection due to their looks, race, ethnicity, colour, and more. When this kind of things happen to us, we might start to form certain negative opinions against a particular race, ethnic group, or colour. Especially if the person who has rejected us fits into one of the categories mentioned above. We must realize that everybody is not the same and that everyone has their own ways of doing things.

Some individuals can even reject you for no reason at all. If rejection can be genuinely justified, that is a whole different story, but if it is based on one of the above reasons, that is when it becomes a problem. Some community members today are facing rejection in one way or the other from other communities; these negative practices cannot move people forward.

Not everyone has the strength to deal with this kind of situation. Some might take it lightly, while others may not, which can easily take them off track and make them use wrong coping strategies. People that can take it lightly are those who believe in the possibility of things getting better and with positive mindsets. The ones who could not take it lightly are those who have less strength and resiliency. That is why we all must be careful when we make such decision because it can negatively change people's lives forever.

Good coping strategy

It is said that every rejection in life is a redirection to greater things. This is one of my personal and favourite quotes. When we are rejected or denied access to certain things in life, we always feel dejected and unhappy with ourselves. It is understandable and natural to feel that way, but what we should understand is that it is not the end of the world. All we need to do is to know our worth, for when we know our worth and what we can do, what other people think of us does not matter.

We should always have a positive and open mindset and believe that if one door closes, another one opens. Many doors are going to be shut against you; many doors are going to be slammed in your face; many people are going to tell you NO, but let their NO be your power, your strength, and your motivator. It is not advisable for people to get stressed when being rejected—knowing who you are is more significant than the thoughts of others.

We should not try to control how others look at us or the opinion they form about us. Oftentimes, some of them just reject others for no reason. When you start to see rejection as an opportunity of attaining greater heights, your stress level will become extremely low, and accepting rejection in good faith will automatically make you stronger and more resilient.

Chapter Thirty-One
DEPRESSION

DEPRESSION IS ANOTHER intense stressor that could inflict a significant amount of damage on anyone passing through it. Depression is caused by excessive stress from the adversities of life. Many people think depression only shows when we are bitter, crying, sad, angry or aggressive over every little thing, but oftentimes depression is also when we do things pretentiously. For example, dancing when we do not want to, crying when we do not feel like, smiling when we do not want to. Doing things we do not want to do also reveals depression—this is the kind of depression that is not always obvious because it is occurring through pretentious activities.

Depression affects parts of the brains which can later result in different kinds of mood swings. It is quite difficult to actually figure out causes of depression as it depends on the individual and the level of stress they can take. Most times it is through excessive, intense stress that depression can occur. It is rare for people to go into depression right away from whatever they are going through. It takes time to graduate from intense stress to depression.

Depression is more common in women than in men; women have a higher percentage of depression than the men. In the world today, one in every five women and one in every ten men suffer from depression at some point in their lives. Depression has different levels, and the worst of all is the major depression level. It is harder for people who have major depression to recover than people who just have regular depression.

The earlier depression is dealt with the better because at the major stage, many individuals feel that all they want to do is take their own life. Remember, intense stress can graduate into major depression, and during that integration, many things can happen to your body. You may have gone through fatigue, pains in your body, inability to sleep, mood swings, post-traumatic stress disorder (PTSD), changes in appetite, and many more symptoms. So, depression not only affects you mentally and psychologically, it also affects you physically.

Good coping strategy

Most times when people are in the early stages of depression, they tend to manage it with minimal effort, but when it gets to the major stage they need more effort and support to be able to deal with the situation. Depression is not something you should ignore or deal with alone; there are resources you could use to better your situation. When we are dealing with extreme stress, depressive symptoms may start to emerge—and when those symptoms emerge, we should try to use the good coping strategies we already know.

First, you should acknowledge what caused you to get depressed. Draft those things out and outline the number of times you feel depression daily. Familiarize yourself with the things that trigger your depression, and try resisting it anytime those depressive thoughts strike your mind. Try to engage yourself with the things that you enjoy doing, both indoors and outdoors. When we are happy, our immune system will become stronger and create natural antidepressants in our bodies, which will give us the strength to resist the effects of our depression.

As well, we can start to explore other areas of interest because the more we discover and engage ourselves with things that make us happy, the faster we will recover from depression. You should look for positive reasons to live your life; think of the things that give you joy and not those that bring sadness or bad memories. Never think of giving up on yourself—think in terms of fight or flight. Fight for yourself—when we try using the flight response to depression instead, we end up using bad coping strategies which will land us in a deeper mess.

Standing our ground and fighting back with all our strength will deter depression and reduce it drastically. Using the wrong coping strategy or running away from our problems does not make it go away—rather it gives it more strength to reinforce against us. It is not easy to deal with depression, but you shouldn't give in easily to it. When those thoughts of giving up come to your mind, think of positive reasons to live, as mentioned above.

Always remember that extreme stress changes into depression, and when we fight it in those early stages, depression is likely not to occur. If at any time you feel things are not improving and you have exhausted all your good coping skills as indicated above, you can seek the services of a counsellor or psychologist who could help you further in dealing with your situation.

Chapter Thirty-Two
HAVING A BAD DAY

HAVING A BAD day is another stressor that can have a huge impact on our daily lives. Little things can trigger people to start having a bad day. A bad day could start from when you leave your home in the morning. It could start from things like greeting someone in the morning; how they respond to you could trigger you to start having a bad day. The person or people might not notice how you perceive their response or responses. People are created differently; the way you will perceive certain things might be different from the way others will perceive it.

Sometimes we stress over things that are not even true. Just because we read different meaning to something does not mean it is true. A bad day could start from a single phone call from a family member, or a friend notifying you of a bad situation, or hearing something that someone has said about you. Hearing things that are not pleasant to our ears can trigger and stress us out. Misinformation and gossip in our workplace can also make us have a bad day too.

Imagine a co-worker telling you that another co-worker told them you have a bad breath, body odour, or that you are not competent for your job. This will certainly trigger your mood and affect your performance throughout that day.

Another thing that could cause a bad day is receiving a call from your child's teacher notifying you about your child's low grades and bad performance in class. Hearing of your child not doing well in school can negatively impact your good day and make it a bad one. Sometimes, bad jokes with friends, family members, and colleagues at work can also trigger your mood and make you have a bad day, so it's important to be aware of the jokes we crack with family, friends, and other people around us.

Good coping strategy

Every day we all go through different situations that can easily trigger our moods and feelings. The way you start your day is very important because it could determine how the rest of the day will be for you. People perceive information in different ways. What might get me upset might not get you upset. When we are dealing with people, we should first study who they are and try to learn how they respond to certain things.

Some people's emotions can easily be hurt by common jokes, and those jokes can negatively impact their feelings throughout that day. That is why it is imperative to observe others before engaging with them. There are several things you can do to cope with stress when having a bad day. The first thing you can do is to disconnect your thoughts from that thing that caused you to start having a bad day; try not thinking about it.

Another thing is to try to interpret different meanings to what was said or done to you by intentionally giving positive meanings to them. I know this is not an easy task, but it is possible to achieve. The aim is to try to change your negative thoughts into positive ones. Always remember that some people don't often realize how hurtful their words are to you. They may not actually mean to hurt you with their words—you just read a different meaning into it.

This is not to make excuses for them; it is simply to throw more light on people's behaviour and how people can read different meanings to certain things. Some people just say whatever comes out of their mouth, considering them to be mere words, not realizing that those words can hurt like the piercing of a sword. When you come across such people, try to interpret their words in more positive ways than the negative ways. To effectively use this strategy, you must first forgive them.

Another thing you can do to eliminate your stress when having a bad day is to take a step back, look at the situation from different angles, and take deep breaths. When you step back and take deep breaths, this will calm your anger and reduce your stress. Most times, stepping back will allow you to reenergize yourself, and when you take deep breaths, you can feel the relief right away after each breath. Do not just take deep breaths—make sure you take those deep breaths slowly and up to five times, five seconds in and five seconds out. Please understand that taking deep breaths might not completely eliminate all the stress in you, but it will definitely reduce it to a controllable level. This also depends on the individual.

The other thing you could do is to break things down—thoughtfully explore what is happening around the world and compare them to what is happening to you. When you do this, you will find that your situation is even better than the situations that many people are in around the world. Ask yourself these questions: Is my case really the worst? Is this really worth stressing over? These are some of the questions you should ask yourself before drowning in those negative thoughts that bring you stress. The more positive thoughts you have in your mind, the better your immune system, as well as your physical and mental health. Engross yourself in more positivity by believing that things are going to get better.

Chapter Thirty-Three
LOW GRADES

LOW GRADES IN school is another stressor that affects the lives of many students. We all know what it feels like to work so hard in our academics and end up getting low grades. This experience can be degrading and can make students lose confidence in themselves. Low grades can make parents lose confidence in their children too. Any time a child finds out that their parents have lost confidence in them, they in turn will start to lose confidence in themselves. It takes encouragement and constant support from parents to help their children overcome their loss of confidence.

Some people can have good grades in some courses and bad grades in others they do not fully understand. Let us, for example, consider students who have dyslexia. Dyslexia is one of the disorders that involves difficulty in reading or interpreting words. When someone is dyslexic, it does not really mean that they are not intelligent; it simply means that they are having difficulties understanding how to read or interpret letters. Such students may not do very well in English and will end up having a low grade in that particular course.

Most dyslexic students are highly intelligent in other areas of their studies. If you look at many successful people in the world today, you will see they experienced dyslexia in one way or the other when in school at some point in their lives. People like Whoopi Goldberg, Steven Spielberg, Anderson Cooper, Muhammed Ali, Jennifer Aniston, Tom Cruise, Albert Einstein just to mention a few. To be dyslexic is not a life sentence because at some point that condition can change to something positive in your life. When students are not doing well in few courses, it does not mean they cannot do well in others. Young students of today may not understand why they get low grades; when they do not understand the reason why their grades are low, they can begin to stress out.

Understanding and identifying dyslexia at an early stage is key to dealing with the disorder properly. After finding out your child is dyslexic you can seek the resources and assistance you need to help to make them successful in their studies. Low grades can have a negative impact on students whose teachers and parents have no idea of what dyslexia is about. As parents, we must perform our own duties and observations of our children who are not getting good grades in school. We must ask them questions in order to get information from them. We need this information to be able to get them the help they need to improve in their studies.

This is not to say that all dyslexic situations are the same. In some cases, it could be hereditary from the mother or father. Getting frustrated or stressed out is quite common with young children when they are experiencing low grades after so much hard work at school. The earlier proper solutions are sought, the better for the child.

Some students may not have dyslexia and still not do well in school. Some of them do not want to pay attention in class, and some even skip classes. When a child starts to skip classes, stops doing their homework, or gets defensive and agitated when confronted about their academics, you will know that things are not right.

Parents should find out what is really wrong with their children if they notice any changes in their behaviour or attitude. Sometimes their behaviour is simply influenced by their circle of friends. Students should not be left alone to deal with the situation on their own; they need assistance to cope with the stress of low grades. If they are left to deal with the situation alone, they are likely to use the wrong coping strategies to do so.

Another thing that is imperative is to make our child our close friend so that whenever they are going through any stress, they can easily share it with us. That is why constant communication with them is extremely important.

Some parents make their children fear them, but when they are afraid of you, they will not share their problems with you—they will end up sharing it with the wrong people or will start using the wrong coping strategy to manage their stress. Let your children see you as a solution and not an additional problem.

Good coping strategy

Coping with the stress of low grades in school may be easy for some students and difficult for others. When a student's grades are high in school, they tend to continue to do well unless they backslide in one way or the other in their studies. When they are encouraged with their good performance in school, they tend to improve more and more and will continue to do well, but when their effort in not recognized, they are likely to backslide.

Except for dyslexic students, other students who may have low grades in class should examine themselves to determine the kind of life they are living. They should check their circle of friends, how many times they study after school, and how often they pay attention in class. Students should not stress too much over low grades. It's not a life sentence that we should allow to be stuck in our thoughts or influence our ways of doing things.

There are things parents should do to bridge those gaps. Try to evaluate your child, and figure out what you've missed doing in their life. Look to the future and forget about their past low grades; do not use your child's academic struggles against them. This is not to say that you are encouraging your child to have low grades, but as parents, your child's low grades should not be your main concern. Instead, concern yourself with what needs to be fixed to make sure there is improvement in their next semester or term. Try to identify their weaknesses and resolve those areas in which they struggle, and apply more efforts to rebuild their strength and capacity for studying.

Low grades have made intelligent students quit school or drop out of courses they were once in love with due to one singular error. Students should be encouraged to always present their difficult situation and setbacks to their parents, guardians, teachers, or even their classmates. With one or two suggestions from these people, they are likely to do better next time. It is highly recommended for young students or adults to study together with their classmates or peers; that way, each of them in the group can share different ideas and tactics to do better in class.

Help your child to be comfortable and calm with what they have learned so they can apply their knowledge to their next exam. Parents should encourage their child to always read every question carefully before answering it in exam. If for any reason they do not understand the question after reading it twice or not know the answer to the question, they should not get stuck on it—they should move on to other questions and answer them. When they have finished answering the questions they understand, then they can go back to those they did not understand earlier. When they eventually return to the challenging questions, they will be surprised to see how easy they will be for them. This is the best logic to use when writing a test or an exam.

Sometimes, when we have tension within us, we are likely to see and understand things differently, but once the tension reduces, our brain and body chemistry work better. After we are calm, the things that were initially difficult for us will become much easier. During these times of difficulties and low-grade stress, we maybe be tempted to use bad coping strategies that will be detrimental to our health. If we can resist temptation for the first couple of days and apply the good coping strategies mentioned above, we will definitely overcome it and do well on our next exams or tests without using any of the bad coping strategies.

Chapter Thirty-Four
LOSS OF A GAME

MANY INDIVIDUALS STRESS a lot when they lose their favourite game. Sports games can bring unity and peace among people—and can also make people fight and dislike one another. Losing our favourite game can be incredibly stressful to us, especially to some people who are extremely passionate about games. When we lose a game, we start experiencing bitterness, anger, aggressiveness, and sleeplessness. The stress of losing a game does not only happen to the players; it also affects their spectators. There are some supporters who feel more pain and frustration more than the actual players of the game.

These supporters never miss any game; they dedicate their time and spend their money to make sure they at the venue before the game kicks off. They show more commitment to the game than other supporters, and when their team loses any game, they always experience that extreme stress which could ruin their entire day. These supporters are sometimes called sports fanatics. There are cases where spectators become really violent after a game loss and fight their rival's supporters; sometimes they even destroy property, causing millions of dollars' worth of damage, all because of the stress of losing the game.

Some spectators go as far as harming or even killing the other team's supporters just because they lost the game. When some teams are on the brink of losing a game, they sometimes bring out their frustrations on their opponents by fighting them at the slightest opportunity. Some players even attack referees and other game officials when they lose a game. Other people who experience intense stress during games are those players who made the mistakes that led to their team losing the game. It affects them big time because they will be looking at themselves as the black sheep that caused their team to lose the game.

Sometimes supporters will violently go after these players to make life more miserable for them. This happened in the case of Andrés Escobar in Colombia, and other similar cases of players being attacked or killed after making a mistake in a game that resulted in them losing. Escobar was also nicknamed "the gentleman" because he was a good player known for his calmness and gentleness when playing a game. But when he made that mistake on that fateful day, all his previous good deeds were forgotten and never put into consideration before one of his team's supporters attacked him. Many supporters labelled him a traitor and looked for ways to execute him. Eventually, he was trailed and brutally murdered for a simple mistake he made in a game.

Escobar believed his error was just a mistake; he expected everyone to understand, but they never did. Some of his team's supporters took it the wrong way and finally assassinated him. His team's supporters failed to realize that Escobar was passionate about the game too and could not have possibly and intentionally made such a huge mistake. The above story is to show you the extent supporters can go to when they lose their favourite game—and also to make you understand what the stress of losing a game can make people do. This is not to make excuses for supporters or to justify their wrongdoings or actions because no one has the right to take what they cannot give: life. This is just to illustrate the extent and extra miles people can go after losing the game they love.

On the other hand, it is also difficult for young children when they lose a game because most of them will not easily understand the concept of games. Most children will not understand that a game is about winning or losing, and what most children are interested in is winning the game. Some children may understand that concept, and some might not understand it. Those that may not understand it can go for days or even weeks still feeling the stress of the defeat; however, the ways people react after losing a game are different and varies. Some people respond to game loss calmly while some act on the loss aggressively and violently.

Good coping strategy

Losing your favourite game should not be the end of the world. You must learn how to derive joy and happiness from the victory of others. You must understand that games are about winning or losing, and you should develop that habit of having an open mind towards every game. When people are too passionate and close-minded about sports games, and then lose, the outcome of the game can negatively impact them. Sports games should be seen as the promoter of love, peace, togetherness, and unity in our society.

When a player makes a mistake in a game, they should not be labelled a black sheep, and their fans should not attack them. Each time people make mistakes, they learn from it, and from their lessons they can do better next time. Let us always see mistakes as part of a game instead of stressing over the lost. There are cases where coaches tear their players apart by yelling at them after making mistake in a game; it should not be that way because blaming them is going to stress them more and get them more confused. And when they are confused, they will not perform well anymore in the game. Coaches should show more support and empathy when confronting players about their mistakes in a game.

Whenever a player makes mistake, they need encouragement; that encouragement refocuses them in the game, which will make them perform well in the game. It is okay to cry, and it is okay to be bitter after losing a game, but it is not good to be angry and violent just because you lost a game. Prepare ahead of time before the game by acknowledging that it is just a game and not a battlefield. Share your support among all the teams involved in the game competition so that when any one of them wins, you can share in their victory. Learn to make the actual game your centre of focus and not the teams involved.

Now, let us explore how children can cope after losing a game. Whenever your child loses a game, do not yell at them; they are already in a bad mood. Instead, give them words of encouragement and let them learn from their mistakes. It is okay if they cry over a lost game; let them pour out their frustrations through tears. Adults cry over game loss too, so if children do the same thing is not a big deal.

The worst thing you can do to your child is to force them to suppress feelings of defeat inside of them. Suppressing these feelings may trigger tantrums. Never put your child down just because their team lost a game—always be the source of support and encouragement whenever they are experiencing the stress of a game loss.

If possible, do not talk about the loss to your child until they have a chance to rest, eat, and freshen up. When they are relaxed, they will be able to comprehend whatever you will tell them about the game loss. Start by commending them for their efforts; let them know the areas in which they did well before you discuss the areas in which they did wrong. Ask them what they have learned from the game's defeat, and teach them how they can improve in their next game.

Chapter Thirty-Five
BREAKUP

RELATIONSHIP BREAKUP IS another stressor affecting many people, especially young people in our society; there is a reason why they are most vulnerable in this area.

When a child hits their teens, there is always the possibility of them crushing on someone they like. And that someone could be their classmate, neighbour, or somebody they came across in one way or the other. Whether they are a boy or girl, teenagers easily trust people—especially the one they are crushing on; they always believe that when they are together with their crush nothing on this earth can come between them.

If a breakup happens between them, that is when they experience stress. As they are not yet fully emotionally mature, that stress can impact virtually everything they do.

Breaking up with someone you love wholeheartedly can be disheartening and stressful. Of course, breakups affect fully grown adults too, but since breakups impact the emotions so profoundly, it is more keenly felt among young people, who are more sensitive during their teenage years.

A breakup is incredibly challenging to cope with, especially when you are all alone. Breaking up with someone you do not love is much easier to cope with, but breaking up with someone you really love can be heartbreaking, stressful, and difficult. The breakup might make you feel that you are never going to heal and that your heart will never stop bleeding, and that you will continue to have sleepless nights, but there are things you can do to make the breakup process easier.

Good coping strategy

When somebody we love breaks up with us, there are emotional and psychological drains attached to it. The first thing we need to do is to talk about it to other people close to us. Going through emotional stress after a breakup is not as easy as people think. Anyone that has experienced a breakup always finds it difficult to trust again, and when they refuse to trust again, it will even affect them more. Some of the best ways to cope with the stress of a breakup is to forgive those who broke up with us, learn to live without them, and learn to love again—as well as learning to trust again.

When we stop loving or trusting after a breakup, we enslave ourselves to the memory of that person who broke up with us. That is why some people's new relationships don't work: they bring the garbage from their previous relationship to the new one and continue to live in their past. Their impulses and the ways they do things will now be impacted by that previous relationship. When we break up with our boyfriend, girlfriend, husband or wife, allow their memories to stay in our past. It is only when we do not put them in our past that they begin to affect our future relationships.

Breaking up is never easy, even if you are the one initiating the end of the relationship. Immediately after a breakup, try to find yourself again. Finding yourself means trying to live well again, trying to love yourself or someone else again, and trying to trust someone again. This is not to say that this whole process is easy to follow, but if we work towards it, it is possible to achieve. Try to do things you have always wanted to do—see your breakup as an opportunity to do things you couldn't do before. For example, you can go to new places and make new friends. Do not isolate yourself, and do not transfer the disappointment and frustration from your former relationship to your new relationship and the new people you meet.

Always give the new people you meet the benefit of the doubt because the only way the true identity of people is revealed to you is through your inner feelings and with time. If you are not able to cope using the above strategies, you could seek the help of a professional counsellor or therapist who will walk you through effective channels to better deal with your stress.

Chapter Thirty-Six
DEBT

MANY PEOPLE GO through stress when they are sinking in debt. People are brought up differently, which is why some feel comfortable being in debt while others do not. To some, it's okay to be in debt; it will never bother them; for others, it's a big burden. It all comes down to the kind of heart they have, how they were nurtured, and the amount of stress they can take. Many people do not feel comfortable owing money to the banks, lenders, family members, or friends. These people easily go through stress when they are indebted to people.

Stress usually gets worse when all you have is at risk because of your debt. Many families face this situation every day; that is why it is important to be prepared and capable of doing things before you need to do them. When you do things because your neighbour did it, you are not only attracting stress to yourself, you are attracting it to your entire family as well because everyone in the family will suffer the outcome of your decision.

Debt has done a whole lot of bad things to relationships and marriages. The stress of debt has broken so many peaceful homes and families. As the saying goes, "What touches the eyes touches the nose as well," which means that being in debt will affect not just you but your entire family. If the stress of debt is not well handled, it could develop into depression, which could then lead to suicidal thoughts and end disastrously.

Many couples have broken up because of the debt incurred during their wedding ceremonies or other family events. It is tragic to go into debt after borrowing money to finance your wedding, impacting the marriage by that same debt, then ending up in separation or divorce while still trying to pay off the debt. This affects so many marriages and relationships today. The earlier people start learning how to sew their coats according to their sizes, the better for every one of them.

Good coping strategy

We live in a competitive world, which drives many people to live above their means. Many families are sinking in debt today because they are trying to live their lives to please others. Sinking in debt is like trying to walk up on an escalator that is going down. One of the methods to use in coping with the stress of debt is to learn to live your life below your means.

There is a quote that reflects how some people enslave

themselves mentally just to please others: "The greatest prison anyone can live in is the fear of what others think of them." This quote reveals how far some people will go when stressing over what others think of them. Stressing ourselves over things we cannot control is not worth doing. You should be more concerned about yourself and not how people see you or what they think of you.

When it comes to avoiding or managing debt, all you need to do is learn to live below your means. When you live below your means, you will be able to save up to buy the things you need as well as for other potential investment opportunities that may arise. Cut down on the things you do not need, focus on your present situation and your future, and forget about everything in your past. Your focus now should be how to repay your debt by working out a repayment plan with your bank or lender. That repayment plan will not only reduce your stress level—it will also give you peace of mind.

Avoid unnecessary outings, stick to your budget, live within your means, stay positive, avoid extravagance, take care of your properties to enable them last long, create a monthly bill repayment plan, pay your monthly minimum, at least, and buy only the things you need. Debt can limit the ways we enjoy our lives, but managing stress using the right coping strategy will give us the chance to live a more meaningful life.

Chapter Thirty-Seven
ADDITIONAL GOOD COPING STRATEGIES

ANY TIME YOU are stressing over your problems, you should always take them to God in prayer. When we pray with faith about our problems, we are asking God to take total control of our situation. When God speaks to your situation, his words will never return to him void, nor will your situation remain the same. If at any time you feel like shedding tears for the pain you are going through, there is nothing wrong with that. It's okay to cry. It's okay to be scared. But giving up shouldn't be an option.

Stress makes us grow stronger and more resilient and is not a death sentence. You should always be optimistic about your situation no matter what you are going through because when we have positive thoughts about ourselves, positive things are likely to happen to us. Make friends with people who support your dreams and not those who undermine them. Never associate yourself with people who make you feel alone; make friends with those who positively boost your spirit, and stay away from those who bring out the worst in you. Always remember the good times you have had in your life and do not dwell on the unpleasant experiences.

Do not get mad at your problems because if you get mad at something, you cannot find solutions. Anger does not yield good fruit; it always attracts negativity. When we get angry, we lose our minds, and whatever decisions we make in those moments are always wrong. When we stress and worry too much, all we can think about are things that get us more worried because negativity attracts negativity. Sometimes most of the things we worry and stress about end up not happening at all because they were only in our imagination.

Never push yourself past your point of comfort in your dealings in life; when you do that you are inviting stress and worry to yourself. Try using mindful meditation, self-relaxation, and yoga to help reduce your stress. Playing good music is one of the good ways people cope with stress. When we play the music we really love, it makes us forget the things that stress us out, so it is important to play our favourite music or listen to that radio channel or watch TV programs that makes us happy.

Spend time in nature. Sometimes when we see the beautiful things God has made, it gives us joy and hope that life is worth living. Do not live for the approval of others, and always do the things that give you joy and happiness. Eat good fruits like grapefruit, oranges, and other citrus fruits that are rich in vitamin C; these fruits have been proven to help reduce stress. Another thing that we should understand is that people can make us laugh, make us smile, and make us feel good, but they cannot make us happy because happiness comes from within.

We are responsible for our own happiness, just as anyone else is responsible for theirs, so we should not base our happiness on other people—we should base it on God and ourselves. If at some point you feel like your stress level is out of control and you are constantly worrying every day, try to limit the time you worry about those things each day—and do this on a daily basis. With time, you will get used to these limits on stress, and from there you can start reducing your allowable stress time step by step until the time wears off and you do not have to stress anymore. We should all understand that life is unpredictable; sometimes it smiles at us and other times it frowns at us. The earlier we understand the concept of ups and downs about life, the better for all of us.

Chapter Thirty-Eight

EFFECTS OF BAD COPING STRATEGIES

Cigarette use

MANY PEOPLE ENGAGE themselves in different negative coping strategies when going through stress. Some people smoke cigarettes to cope with their stress. Smoking cigarettes can make you temporarily forget the stress, but it does not take it away permanently. As soon as you take the last puff of a cigarette and toss the butt, your stress will immediately resume duty on you. Stress cannot be permanently eliminated always because stress is a response to different situations, and we must consistently deal with it before it fades away with time.

Engaging yourself in such habits to alleviate your stress does not help—rather, it makes it worse. Cigarettes destroy your body and do not do anything good for it. Cigarettes, for example, have over two hundred chemicals in it which can trigger lung cancer and other deadly diseases. Your lungs are the first target by the chemicals from the cigarettes you smoke. Immediately your lungs are affected, and you will begin to experience the following: coughs, sneezing, wheezing, asthma, and difficulty breathing.

These symptoms are just the beginning of your ordeal; it's nothing compared to what you will suffer later when you will be diagnosed with emphysema, pneumonia, lung cancer, stroke, or chronic obstructive pulmonary disease. Smoking can cause cancer almost anywhere in your body, and it does not matter the number of cigarettes you smoke in a day. The fact is that you are smoking cigarettes and they contain hundreds of chemicals that expose you to many health problems. Please look at the below YouTube documentary to see things for yourself - https://www.youtube.com/watch?v=Y18Vz51Nkos

Alcohol use

Alcohol use is another negative method that people go to when coping with their stress. There are numerous chemicals in alcohol that can destroy many vital organs in your body. Excessive alcohol consumption can affect your liver, kidneys, and other vital organs in your body as well as the ways your brain functions. There are a whole lot of negative things alcohol does to your body, and these disruptions affect how you function on your day-to-day life.

These disruptions could also affect your mood,

behaviour, and your ability to think clearly. Constant drinking of alcohol can lead you to many health challenges like diabetes, diarrhea, stroke, bloating, gassiness, ulcer, hemorrhoids, digestive problems, and other various health issues. When you drink alcohol frequently to cope with stress, there are common areas in the body where you can easily develop cancer—your lungs, throat, liver, colon, and esophagus, for example.

This is not to say that cancer cannot start anywhere in your body, but these are the key areas they are likely to start from. Many people think that it is only when you drink a lot of alcohol that it starts affecting you. The fact is that the effects start right away from when you take your first sip. Alcohol does more harm to women than men because in women it takes more time to process due to other many additional vital organs in them that men do not have.

Alcohol consumption is always bad for the body, and this is just a warning that the longer alcohol stays in our body the more damage it does. On that note, women are more exposed to more damage than the men. This is not to encourage men to continue drinking alcohol; the bottom line is that alcohol consumption is bad for everyone, regardless of how we think we can manage it, or the gender it affects more. Seeing is believing—please, look at the below YouTube documentary to see things for yourself - https://www.youtube.com/watch?v=hwZPb1uQqmY

Hard drug use

In addition to the bad coping strategies mentioned above, there are several other dangerous drugs, like cocaine, that people use to cope with their stress. The question is, are these negative coping strategies really helping us solve our problems? Obviously, the answer is no. There are several hard drugs out there we can elaborate on but let us look at one of them. Before we discuss the effects of cocaine on our bodies, let us look at the things cocaine is made of. Cocaine alone is made with the most dangerous chemicals on earth. You should take a look at documentaries on YouTube and other social media platforms on how cocaine is processed.

To start with, we will discuss the contents of cocaine. After this analysis, you will definitely change your mind against using this substance to cope with stress. Here is a list of some of the things cocaine contains: Coca leaves, fuel and gas, baking soda, cement powder, caustic soda, potassium salt, battery acids, and other deadly chemicals. Cocaine can do lots of negative things to your body: it can limit or hinder your ability to smell things right; it can affect your heartbeat by reducing or increasing the rate; it can make your nose bleed profusely; it can block your lungs by limiting its air flow.

Cocaine is highly addictive to the extent that whenever you experience a little stress, you crave cocaine. It is not good or advisable to even smell cocaine, much less inhale it. One thing we should keep in mind is that cocaine is quite easy to start using, but to stop it is where the problem is. Millions of people out there sob and have regrets; if they had known that cocaine was this addictive and destructive, they would not have even got close to it. It is only through education and awareness of the nature of this substance (and others) that we can gain knowledge and insight of how dangerous these bad coping strategies can affect our health.

You should always remember that the effects of your

excessive smoking, drinking, and use of hard drugs during your stressful situations may lead you to various health problems like cancers, strokes, heart diseases, respiratory problems, lungs infections, and more which will remain with you even if you have recovered from your stressful situation. That is why it is always wise not to get involved at all with these bad coping strategies, so that you will not have to live a life of regrets at the end. After you may have recovered from your stress, you will now have to deal with one or more of the above illnesses that originated from your bad coping strategies during your stressful period. Please, look at the below YouTube documentary to see things for yourself: https://www.youtube.com/watch?v=7tlwW2DKzlc&has_verified=1

Stress eating

Stress eating is another way people use to cope with their stress. Some people like eating a lot to cope with their stress, forgetting that too much food can take them out of shape or even make them vulnerable to more health problems. Gaining weight is quite easy, but losing it is extremely difficult.

When you constantly eat food to cope with stress, you expose yourself to further health challenges. Eating food every minute of the day should not be part of stress-coping strategies, but some people find solace in this activity when coping with their stress. In some cases, when their stressor is gone, they are already addicted to eating all the time and cannot stop anymore. Some other health issues may have already developed from their excessive eating, and now they have to deal with that new health challenge.

It is imperative to understand what excessive eating can

do to your body and to try avoiding that habit. There is no doubt food is good for the body, but eating it all the time and excessively is a big problem to our health.

Blaming others

Some people resort to blaming others for everything that happens to them, or for their misfortunes. Blaming other people for the mess we created ourselves or the ones that happened naturally is never going to solve our problems. When we blame other people, we are creating room for excuses and denial. We should always accept our faults and mistakes so that we can concentrate on finding lasting solutions to them through the use of the right coping strategies.

Blaming other people for our problems will not make the problems disappear; rather it will worsen our situation, which will give room for bad coping strategies. Accusing or blaming other innocent people for what they did not do is going to trigger their mood and ignite their anger. When that happens, the situation may go from bad to worse for you, which can eventually aggravate your stress level.

If you use one or more of these bad coping strategies, it is not too late to quit them. The earlier you do away with these things, the better for you. We should put all the negative effects of bad coping strategies into consideration so that we can determine to do away with them. One thing to keep in mind: the more we consume these bad chemicals found in cigarettes, alcohol, and hard drugs, the more they destroy us. Eating excessively and blaming others rather than ourselves is not a good thing for us either.

Always remember that we cannot control or stop certain things from happening to us. When those things happen to us, they may mold us, they may alter us, they may shape us, but they do not have to define us. We should do all we can to make sure who we really are remain in us. Problems are part of life; we cannot solve all our problems, but we can handle them according to God's promises in the bible. Our prayer should be: "God grant us the serenity to accept what we cannot change and courage to change the things we can." When we try to change the things that we cannot change, this affects our productivity in life.

Anytime we are in stressful situations, we should always look for things to be grateful for—things like being alive and not dead, not in jail, not in the hospital, not homeless, having life, having food, having clothes, having water, and having health. The list can go on and on for the things we should be grateful for. And remember, around the world there are lots of people born with different afflictions—people who are in much more difficult situations than we can even imagine.

Many are born different and with many life challenges, and they still find something to be grateful for. People are born with Bilateral Amelia, Bilateral Phocomelia, Tetra-Amelia syndrome, Uterus Didelphys, paralysis, diabetes, glaucoma, lamellar ichthyosis, blindness and many other difficult medical conditions, but they still have reasons to be happy and glorify God that at least they have life. Those who have problems with their hands are grateful that they have legs; those who have problems with their legs are grateful that they have hands; and those who have problems all over their bodies are grateful that they have life.

The gift of life is incomparable to worldly things. We should not take what we have for granted because there are many out there who do not have the opportunities we have.

People are dying every single day; some left their home in the morning and did not return. Some people slept at night and woke up with one illness or the other, and some could not wake up at all, so we should always be grateful for our life. Trials make us stronger and a better person. Stop procrastinating in getting closer to God, and embrace him wholeheartedly by doing away with things that are not pleasing to him.

You should always remember that the effects of your excessive smoking, drinking, and use of hard drugs during your stressful situation can lead you to various health problems like cancer, stroke, heart disease, respiratory problems, and lungs infections, which will remain with you even if you have recovered from your stressful condition. That is why it is always wise not to get involved at all in those bad coping strategies, so that you will not have to live a life full of regrets at the end. After your stress may have gone, you will now have to deal with the ailment of those wrong coping strategies during your stressful period.

When you make excuses by hiding behind the shadow of stress to excessively smoke, drink, and use hard drugs, a time will come, after your stress may have gone, when you will then have to deal with the seeds of the illnesses that cigarettes, alcohol, and hard drugs may have planted inside your body, making your life more miserable and extremely stressful.

If you are already using the above bad coping strategies to cope with your stress, it is not too late to make things right by quitting. Do not allow your life to continuously rotate in a stressful circle of stress without end—say no to bad coping strategies now to avoid that repeated circle of stress throughout your lifetime.

Conclusion

STRESS HAPPENS ON a daily basis in our lives. A lot of unpleasant things in this world tend to constantly stress us out and weigh us down. We respond to these stressors in different ways and forms. Some people use good coping strategies while others resign to using bad coping strategies.

Both strategies have different effects on our day-to-day living. The good coping strategies enrich our souls by moving us forward in life, while the bad coping strategies reduce our lifespan by increasing our chances of developing chronic illnesses and diseases that may lead us to death.

Stress is part of life—it is something we cannot completely avoid. Stressing over the things that are inevitable and using wrong coping strategies will do us bad rather than good. Quitting and doing away with these negative coping strategies in good time will not only increase our chances of recovering fully from our stress, it will also give us the hope and opportunity to live a better, longer, and more peaceful life.

Acknowledgements

I am grateful to God for making the writing, editing, and formatting of this book a success.

I thank my mother for bringing me up in the ways of God, and I recognize all she went through when raising me and my siblings. Her struggles, perseverance, and determination to stay by us through thick and thin make her worthy of great honour. I am forever humbled and grateful for her resilience during the stressful situations and storms that she endured throughout her life and ours.

Thanks to my precious immediate family members for the significant roles they played, and how they supported my journey of writing this book.

Thanks to my editor, Ranee Layberry and her team for their roles in making this book achieve its desired purpose.

This is a non-fiction book. All the events described are real; they accurately represent the struggles and stress people go through. The bible verses are extracted from the King James version, both online and hard copy. All other references are authentic past and current events that are happening around the world.

References

Chapters 1, 4

World Cup stunning moments: Andrés Escobar's deadly own goal. *The Guardian*, April 3, 2018. Retrieved August 12, 2020.

Chapter 17

World population review. (2020) Rape statistics by Country online. https://worldpopulationreview.com/country-rankings/rape-statistics-by-country

Chapter 20

King James Bible (2020). King James Bible Online: https://www.kingjamesbibleonline.org

Chapters 25, 26

Nelson, Thomas. (2017) Holy Bible. Nashville, Tennessee: Thomas Nelson.

Chapter 31, 33

Cari Nierenberg. (October 27, 2016). 7 ways

depression differs in men and women https://www.livescience.com/56599-depression-differs-men-women-symptoms.html

Klampak FC. (August 23, 2019). The tragic story of Andrés Escobar. Retrieved July 26 2020, https://www.youtube.com/watch?v=RR-D5VKPdmI

Article: "Famous People with Dyslexia": https://www.readandspell.com/famous-people-with-dyslexia

Chapter 38

DocsOnline (April 15, 2014). "Cocaine Production in Colombia." Retrieved September 13, 2020, via https://www.youtube.com/watch?v=7tlwW2DKzlc&has_verified=1
Unreported World (August 11, 2019). "Indonesia's Tobacco Children." Retrieved September 13, 2020, via https://www.youtube.com/watch?v=BsUAAw2qLB8

Rodrigues, Rickson (December 9, 2019). "Effects of Smoking." Retrieved September 14, 2020, via https://www.youtube.com/watch?v=l26f4f-V4jc

TED-Ed (September 13, 2018). "How Do Cigarettes Affect the Body?" Retrieved September 13, 2020, via https://www.youtube.com/watch?v=Y18Vz51Nkos

Whats Up Dude (January 3, 2017). "How Alcohol Affects the Body." Retrieved August 12, 2020, via https://www.youtube.com/watch?v=hwZPb1uQqmY

Very Well Mind (2020). "Women and the Effects of Alcohol." https://www.verywellmind.com/

women-and-the-effects-of-alcohol-63794#:~:text=%20
Multiple%20Factors%20Affecting%20Women%20
%201%20Liver,increases%20the%20risk%20for%20
breast%20cancer%2C...%20More%20

About the Author

BRIGHT DESTINY OSAIYUWU is a writer, motiva-
tor, philanthropist, inspirator, and security professional.
Bright was born in Edo-state, Nigeria, in the western part
of Africa, and is currently living in Toronto, Canada, with
dual citizenship.

His experiences in life and observations of things happening around the world prompted him to draft out this
book on how people can manage their stress. He had his
early education in Nigeria and post-secondary education
in Canada.

The author's mission is to inspire, motivate, and
encourage his readers and listeners to always be optimistic,
no matter what life throws at them. He believes that positive thinking attracts positive things while negative thinking
attracts negative things.

www.ingramcontent.com/pod-product-compliance
Lightning Source LLC
Chambersburg PA
CBHW060320030426
42336CB00011B/1139